THE GREG DIET COMPANION

Individual Nutrient Rankings

How do your favorite foods rank by each nutrient?

Gregory P. Bullock, Ph.D.

ASIN:

ISBN-13: 978-1546672104

ISBN-10: 1546672109

First Edition

The United States of America

Facebook: https://www.facebook.com/TheGregDiet

Blog: http://thegregdiet.blogspot.com/

Twitter: @The_Greg_Diet

Email: TheGregDiet@gmail.com

TABLE OF CONTENTS

INTRODUCTION

We so often hear opinions on which foods are better. They come from so many various sources that it's hard to know who's right and which sources are the most credible. Beliefs and proclamations on which foods are better usually center on a specific nutrient. Have you ever wondered what foods were highest in each individual nutrient, without having to guess? I wanted definitive and indisputable answers to these questions. To find these answers, I searched the numbers because *numbers don't lie*. For example, we often think of bananas as being *high in potassium*. But did you know that many herbs, spices, nuts, vegetables, seafoods... even potato chips, have more potassium than bananas by raw concentration? (See the full list in the Potassium table).

I wanted a one-stop resource that had the answers to what foods were highest and lowest in *every* major nutrient of *all* the common foods, and even some additional nutrition-related information. So I made it myself....

This book is that resource and is the companion to *THE GREG DIET*. I wrote *THE GREG DIET: The Busy Person's Answer To Better Health* to share my practical and successful methods of good health and weight maintenance, as well as other eye-opening information you won't find in other diet books. Besides the diet and workout system, *THE GREG DIET* also contains The Bullock Nutrition Equation – the first equation ever that ranks all foods by nutritional quality, to reveal *how good or bad foods are*. I invented it as a better alternative to the very ambiguous Nutrition Facts labels, which people find very hard to use for choosing foods. The equation works by using all the available nutrition data for any given food to compute one numeric score. These scores can then be used to compare foods (the higher the score, the better and more nutritious the food) as well as suggest how much to consume per day. Mainly, it helps busy people (but really, anyone) make the quickest and smartest food choices.

The Bullock Nutrition Equation is intricate, taking about 5 years (on and off) to develop, and built through a number of steps. After gathering the data on over 350 foods (and inserting it into an Excel spreadsheet table), the next step was converting the raw data into *Raw Ratio Values*, which are essentially arbitrary nutrient concentrations, calculated by dividing the mass of a nutrient (in whatever unit they are given) by its relative serving size mass (grams). (The Raw Ratio

Values, and all other steps, are explained in detail in *THE GREG DIET*).

I originally intended to include these Raw Ratio Values tables in *THE GREG DIET* book, but as you will see, it would have added over 300 additional pages, and I didn't want to inflate the book size by that much. So I gave them their own separate book. These tables are here for reference for those interested in how foods *rank* by individual nutrient concentration. The book gives answers to questions like:

Which food is higher in a specific nutrient?

in case you are trying to eat foods high in a desired nutrient, or avoid foods high in an undesired nutrient, as may be required for specific medical or dietary reasons, perhaps as recommended by your physician. Additionally, I wanted to provide a deeper glimpse at the data and numbers used in The Bullock Nutrition Equation, to make it as transparent as possible.

The values in this book only show what foods are higher in each nutrient. But this book does not say whether a food is high, low, normal, average, good, bad, or any other designation, for that nutrient concentration of a food. If you're looking for answers to those questions, you must seek other resources.

Although this book shows foods ranked by individual nutrients, you should use caution and discretion in *using* this information when choosing foods. Food choices should be made on more than one (or a few) nutrients, thus the purpose of The Bullock Nutrition Equation; read more on *One-Dimensional Thinking* in *THE GREG DIET*. Always consult with your physician for food choices and any dietary changes.

Each food listing was taken directly from my table of data from The Bullock Nutrition Equation; therefore the listings are the same as they are shown in The BNE Food Score Rankings in *THE GREG DIET* book... So for many foods you will see notes in parentheses saying that some nutrient data is missing. It should be noted that the "missing data" does not affect the raw ratio values of other nutrients because each nutrient value is divided by the given relative serving size. The effect that missing nutrient information *does* have is generating *no value* for the respective nutrient raw ratio value. The Bullock Nutrition Equation reads these as "0" because: how can you count something that isn't there? This is different than foods that actually have zero concentration of some nutrients. To prevent any confusion between which foods have a zero concentration of a nutrient and which foods *show* a zero concentration due to missing data, any raw ratio value of "0.000" for any food, no matter the reason, has been omitted from these tables.

There are a few extra tables provided in this book that were calculated in my work, but were ultimately not used for The Bullock Nutrition Equation. However, I have provided them here as a courtesy to anyone interested in them, and, in the least, to save you the work of calculating them yourself. They include:

- Calories / Serving Size
- Ratio of Total Omega-3 Fatty Acids to Total Omega-6 Fatty Acids
- Protein (g) / Serving Size (g)
- Protein (g) / Calories

The foods that make up the Averages (shown throughout as "Avg.") are listed in The Explanation of The Bullock Nutrition Equation in *The Greg Diet* book.

Finally, a lot of data was taken and transcribed for The Bullock Nutrition Equation, so it is possible that some are wrong due to human error in the transcribing process. If you think you have discovered any such errors, please alert me via email at TheGregDiet@gmail.com. Below is a legend of some abbreviations used in the tables to follow.

Legend

IU – International Unit

g – grams

mg – milligrams, which are one thousandth of a gram

ug – micrograms, which are one thousandth of a milligram, and one millionth of a gram.

SS – Serving size, in grams

Calories / Serving Size

Please note that "calories" represents total calories, and are not distinguished by the different *type of calories* (carbs, fat or protein).

Calories per Serving Size	Food
9.020	Lard (No Trans Fat Data)
8.843	Olive oil (Missing Trans Fat Data)
8.843	Palm oil (Missing Trans Fat Data)
8.840	Shortening, industrial, soy (partially hydrogenated) for baking & confections (Missing O3FA Data)
8.839	Sesame oil (Missing Trans Fat Data)
8.839	Canola oil (vegetable oil), low erucic acid rapeseed oil
8.839	Grapeseed oil (vegetable oil) (Missing Trans Fat Data)
8.839	Safflower oil (vegetable oil), salad or cooking, linoleic, (over 70%) (No Trans Fat or O3FA Data)
8.839	Sunflower oil (vegetable oil) (Missing Trans Fat & Phytosterol Data)
8.839	Cottonseed (vegetable oil), salad or cooking (Missing Trans Fat Data)
8.839	Corn oil (vegetable oil), industrial and retail, all purpose salad or cooking
8.839	Soybean oil, salad or cooking (Missing Phytosterol Data)
8.839	Shortening, vegetable, industrial, soy (partially hydrogenated), all purpose
8.839	Vegetable shortening, household, composite
8.761	Peanut oil, salad or cooking (No Trans Fat or O3FA Data)
8.619	Coconut oil (Missing Trans Fat & O3FA Data)
7.182	Macadamia nuts, dry roasted, w/out salt
7.177	Mayonnaise, soybean oil, w/ salt (salad dressing)
7.172	Butter, salted (No Trans Fat Data)
7.159	Macadamia nuts, dry roasted, with salt
7.140	Margarine, industrial, non-dairy, cottonseed, soy oil (partially hydrogenated), for flaky pastries
7.140	Mayonnaise, Arby's (Missing Vitamin Data)
7.100	Pecans, dry roasted, no salt
6.556	Brazil nuts, dried, unblanched
6.538	Walnuts, USDA A259, A257
6.316	Avg. Nuts
6.220	Margarine (vegetable oil spread, 70% fat, soybean & partially hydrogenated soybean, stick)

5.880	Peanut butter, smooth, USDA Commodity
5.849	Peanuts, dry roasted, no salt, all types
5.820	Sunflower Seeds, hulled, dry roasted, no salt
5.777	Dark chocolate candies, 60-69% cacao solids (Missing Vitamin Data)
5.748	Almonds, USDA A256, A264
5.737	Cashews, dry roasted, no salt
5.707	Pistachio nuts, dry roasted, no salt
5.650	Cheese-flavor puffs or twists, corn-based
5.650	Cheetos Crunchy cheese-flavored snacks (No O3, 6FA Data)
5.500	Beef sticks, smoked (No Trans Fat Data)
5.471	Potato chips, plain, salted
5.440	Pork-skins, plain
5.410	Sesame sticks, wheat-based, salted
5.410	Chocolate-flavored hazelnut spread (No Trans Fat Data)
5.351	Milk chocolate candies (No Trans Fat Data)
5.340	Flaxseed
5.330	Bacon (pork), cured, cooked, pan-fried
5.270	Popcorn, regular butter flavor, microwave, made w/ partially hydrogenated oil (Missing Fats Data)
5.250	Poppy seed
5.250	Nutmeg, ground (Missing O3FA Data)
5.190	Banana chips
5.182	Corn chips, extruded, plain
4.980	Tortilla chips, plain, white corn
4.940	Pepperoni, pork, beef
4.920	Ritz Crackers, Nabisco (Missing Vitamin Data)
4.920	Tortilla chips, plain, yellow corn (Missing Vitamin Data)
4.910	FritoLay Sun Chips, Multi-grain snack, original flavor
4.900	Chia seeds, dried (Missing Sugar and Vitamin Data)
4.752	Candy bar, Snickers (King Size)
4.750	Mace, ground (Missing Data)
4.690	Mustard seed, yellow
4.512	Soybeans (aka soy nuts) mature, dry roasted (Missing Sugar and Vitamin Data)
4.460	Pumpkin/Squash Seeds, dry roasted, no salt (Missing Vitamin & Se Data)
4.370	Ramen noodle soup, chicken flavor, dry

4.330	Cinnamon Toast Crunch cereal, ready-to-eat, General Mills
4.310	Popcorn, caramel-coated without peanuts
4.310	Parmesan cheese, grated (No Trans Fat Data)
4.180	Granola bar, soft, uncoated, chocolate chip
4.160	Peanut Butter Cap'n Crunch, Quaker
4.071	Salami, dry or hard, pork (No Trans Fat Data)
4.070	Lucky Charms, General Mills
4.070	Post Honey Bunches of Oats w/ Almonds (Missing Data)
4.063	Whey protein powder (Low Data)
4.030	Cheddar cheese (No Trans Fat Data)
4.020	Popcorn, microwave, 94% fat free
4.020	Cap'n Crunch, Quaker
4.020	Cap'n Crunch with Crunch Berries, Quaker
4.000	Cocoa Puffs, General Mills
3.990	Cake, snack cakes, crème-filled, chocolate with frosting
3.980	Golden Crisp, Post, Kraft
3.950	Matzo crackers, plain
3.950	Honeycomb cereal, Post, Kraft (low data)
3.930	Froot Loops, General Mills
3.920	Celery seed
3.900	Apple Jacks, Kellogg's
3.891	Oats
3.870	Rice cakes, brown rice, plain
3.870	Popcorn, air-popped
3.870	Sugars, granulated (sucrose)
3.870	Rice Krispies, Kellogg's
3.870	Honey Smacks, Kellogg's
3.813	Corn starch (Missing O3FA Data)
3.810	Cocoa Krispies, Kellogg's (No O3FA Data)
3.803	Swiss Cheese (No Trans Fat Data)
3.800	Brown sugars
3.780	Pretzels, hard, plain, salted
3.780	Corn Pops, Kellogg's
3.750	Kellogg's Nutri-Grain Cereal Bars, fruit-filled
3.750	American cheese, pasteurized, w/out disodium phosphate (No Trans Fat Data)

3.750	Cumin seed
3.700	Kraft macaroni & cheese dinner, original, unprepared (Missing Data)
3.670	Cheerios, General Mills
3.670	Wheaties, General Mills
3.670	Frosted Flakes, Kellogg's
3.660	Puffed Wheat, Quaker
3.640	White flour, white, all-purpose, enriched, bleached
3.620	Pretzels, hard, whole-wheat (Missing Sugar Data)
3.610	Corn Flakes, Kellogg's
3.571	Monterey Jack cheese (Missing Data)
3.569	Potato flour
3.540	Turmeric, ground
3.539	Coconut meat, raw
3.538	Barley (hulled)
3.530	Blue Cheese (No Trans Fat Data)
3.508	Provolone cheese (No Trans Fat Data)
3.455	Avg. Cheese
3.450	Fennel seed (Missing Vitamin & O3FA Data)
3.440	Sausage, Italian, pork, cooked (No Trans Fat Data)
3.422	Cream cheese (No Trans Fat Data)
3.392	Whole wheat flour
3.378	Pretzels, soft
3.370	Anise seed (Missing Sugar, Vitamin, O3FA data)
3.349	Rye
3.342	Avg. Spice
3.330	Caraway seed
3.310	Rosemary, dried (Missing Data)
3.270	Hotdog, Oscar Mayer Wiener, beef frank (No Trans Fat Data)
3.250	Curry powder
3.240	Light mayo (salad dressing)
3.230	Cloves, ground
3.230	Fenugreek seed (Missing Vitamin & O3, 6FA Data)
3.220	Kellogg's Raisin Bran
3.200	Bran Flakes, single brand
3.162	McDonald's French Fries

3.150	Sage, ground
3.140	Chili powder
3.130	Bay leaf (Missing Data)
3.126	Avg. Cased Meat
3.110	Cardamom (Missing Data)
3.100	Spam, Hormel (Missing Data)
3.100	Saffron (Missing Data)
3.060	Oregano, dried
3.041	Honey
3.030	Velveeta cheese, Kraft, pasteurized spread (Missing Data)
3.000	Mozzarella cheese, whole milk (No Trans Fat Data)
2.988	Raisins, seedless
2.980	Coriander seed (Missing Data)
2.950	Tarragon, dried (Missing Data)
2.930	Roll, hard, kaiser
2.890	Paprika
2.860	Agave nectar (Missing Data)
2.838	Avg. Herbs
2.810	High-fructose corn syrup
2.801	T-bone steak, short loin, beef trimmed to 1/8" fat, all grades, broiled
2.790	Cilantro, dried (No O3FA Data)
2.780	Whole wheat bread, prepared from recipe
2.760	Thyme, dried
2.760	Parsley, dried (Missing O3FA Data)
2.750	White pita bread, enriched
2.748	Bagel, plain, unenriched w/ calcium propionate, onion, poppy, sesame (no cream cheese)
2.730	Wheat dinner rolls
2.720	Bologna, chicken, pork, beef
2.710	Hamburger patty, 80/20 ground chuck beef, broiled
2.710	Marjoram, dried
2.660	White bread, commercially prepared (inlcudes soft crumbs)
2.660	Whole wheat pita bread
2.641	Slice of pizza, fast food, pizza chain, 14", cheese topping, regular crust (No Trans Fat Data)
2.630	Allspice (Missing Data)

2.610	Salami, cooked, beef (No Trans Fat Data)
2.609	Syrups, maple
2.550	Black pepper
2.540	Mozzarella cheese, part skim (No Trans Fat Data)
2.530	Dill weed, dried (Missing Data)
2.510	Basil, dried
2.500	Corned beef luncheon meat, beef, cured, canned (No Trans Fat Data)
2.500	Strawberry Jam, Hardee's condiment (Missing Data)
2.470	Whole wheat bread, commecially prepared
2.470	Cinnamon
2.420	Apricot jam and preserves
2.350	Ground turkey, cooked
2.220	Ice cream, soft-serve, french vanilla (No Trans Fat Data)
2.100	Anchovies, European, canned in oil, drained solids
2.070	Ice creams, vanilla (No Trans Fat Data)
1.919	Banquet chicken pot pie, frozen entrée (Missing Data)
1.818	Salmon, Atlantic, wild, cooked in dry heat
1.768	Hummus, home prepared
1.740	Ricotta cheese, whole milk (No Trans Fat Data)
1.733	Soybeans green, boiled, drained, no salt
1.720	Bologna, lebanon, beef (No O3FA Data)
1.670	Egg, whole, cooked, scrambled
1.650	McDonald's barbeque sauce
1.650	Chicken, broilers or fryers, breast, meat only (no skin), roasted
1.640	Chick peas (garbanzo, bengal gram), mature seeds, boiled, no salt
1.620	Beef, eye of round, separable lean only, trimmed to 0" fat, all grades, roasted [cube steak]
1.602	Avocado, raw, commercial varieties
1.579	Spaghetti, cooked, enriched w/out added salt, no sauce
1.547	Swordfish, cooked in dry heat
1.513	Avg. Lean Meat
1.493	Garlic, raw
1.480	Clams, mixed species, cooked in moist heat
1.460	Pastrami luncheon meat, beef, cured (No Trans Fat Data)
1.450	Olives, pickled, canned or bottled, green

1.433	Pinto beans, boiled, no salt, mature
1.430	Pork tenderloin lean, roasted, URMIS 3358
1.420	McDonald's spicy buffalo sauce
1.381	Egg noodles, cooked, enriched
1.379	Banquest Hearty Ones Salisbury Steak Dinner w/ Gravy, Mashed Potatoes and Corn in Seasoned Sauce, frozen meal(Missing Data)
1.370	Oysters, eastern, wild, cooked, moist heat
1.350	Turkey, fryer-roaster, breast meat only, roasted
1.314	Avg. Seafood
1.310	Rosemarry, fresh (Missing Data)
1.297	White rice, long-grain, regular, cooked
1.282	Red snapper, cooked, dry heat
1.281	Turkey, stuffing, mashed potatoes w/ gravy, assorted vegetables, frozen, microwaved
1.280	Tilapia, cooked in dry heat
1.279	Tuna fish, white, canned in water without salt, drained solids
1.271	Kidney beans, red, boiled, no salt, mature seeds
1.229	Lima beans, immature, boiled, drained, no salt
1.228	Parboiled rice, white, long-grain, enriched, cooked
1.220	Weight Watchers Smart Ones Chicken Enchiladas Suiza, Sour Cream w/ Cheese frozen entrée (Missing Data)
1.219	Edamame beans, frozen, prepared
1.200	Quinoa, cooked
1.192	Chick peas (garbanzo, bengal gram), mature seeds, canned
1.190	Millet, cooked
1.174	Avg. Beans & Lentils
1.173	Flounder (sole), cooked in dry heat
1.170	White rice, long-grain, pre-cooked or instant, prepared (Missing O3FA Data)
1.162	Lentils, mature seeds, boiled, no salt
1.160	Whiting, mixed species, cooked in dry heat
1.158	Tuna fish, light, canned in water without salt, drained solids
1.129	Mashed potatoes, home-prepared, whole milk & butter added
1.120	Scallops (bay & sea), steamed
1.108	Brown rice, long-grain, cooked
1.091	Rice noodles, cooked (Missing Sugar & Unsaturated Fat Data)
1.079	Corn, sweet, yellow, boiled, drained, no salt

1.012	Wild rice, cooked
1.010	Thyme, fresh (Missing Data)
1.000	Culver's shrimp cocktail sauce (Missing Vitamin Data)
0.990	Shrimp, mixed species, cooked in moist heat
0.979	Lobster, northern, cooked in moist heat
0.971	White rice, glutinous, cooked
0.971	Ketchup
0.970	Ginger, ground
0.970	Potato, Russet, baked, flesh & skin
0.930	Potato, baked, flesh & skin, no salt
0.908	Black beans, mature seeds, canned
0.900	Sweet potato, baked in skin, no salt
0.890	Banana, raw
0.890	Potato, red, baked, flesh & skin
0.889	Teriyaki sauce, ready-to-serve
0.872	Instant Oatmeal, Quaker, apples & cinnamon prepared w/ boiling water
0.870	Crayfish, mixed species, farmed, cooked in moist heat
0.867	Greek style yogurt 150g=2/3 cup (Missing Data)
0.830	Pomegranate, raw
0.779	Peas, frozen, boiled, drained, no salt
0.721	Cottage cheese, 1% milkfat (No Trans Fat Data)
0.709	Oats, unenriched, boiled, w/out salt
0.689	Grapes, red or green, European type such as Thompson seedless, raw
0.681	Oysters, eastern, wild, raw
0.671	Mustard, prepared, yellow
0.648	Mangos, raw
0.641	New England clam chowder, Campbell's Select (Missing Data)
0.630	Cherries, sweet, raw
0.629	Yogurt, regular low-fat, plain, 12 g protein per 8 oz
0.618	Cream of Wheat, instant, prepared with water and salt
0.602	Pineapple, canned, juice pack, drained
0.601	Grape Juice, canned or bottled, unsweetened
0.598	Milk, whole, 3.25% milkfat
0.591	Grits, corn, white, regular, quick, enriched, cooked with water, with salt

0.588	Greek yogurt
0.570	Blueberries, raw
0.559	Mushrooms, shiitake, cooked, no salt
0.551	Avg. Fruit
0.542	Cranberry juice cocktail, bottled
0.529	Soy sauce (soy & wheat)
0.529	Soy sauce, low sodium (soy & wheat)
0.520	Raspberries, raw
0.520	Apple, raw, with skin A343
0.500	Milk, reduced fat, 2%, added Vit A
0.500	Mustard, Subway, yellow & deli brown (Missing Vitamin Data)
0.497	Pineapple, raw, all varieties
0.480	Horseradish, prepared
0.478	Orange, raw, all commercial varieties
0.462	Apple Juice, canned or bottled, unsweetened
0.440	Spearmint, fresh (Missing Data)
0.435	Coca Cola Classic
0.426	Beets, raw
0.418	Milk, lowfat, 1%, added Vit A
0.417	Pepsi (Missing Data)
0.406	Carrots, raw, USDA A099
0.401	Sprite
0.400	Onion, raw
0.400	Butternut squash, winter, baked w/out salt, sugar or butter
0.393	Papayas, raw
0.389	Peaches, raw
0.371	Avg. Vegetables
0.360	Salsa, USDA Commodity (Missing Sugar and Vitamin Data)
0.352	Snap (green string) beans, boiled, drained, no salt
0.350	Broccoli, boiled, drained, no salt
0.348	Milk, nonfat, Ca fortified
0.343	Cantaloupe, raw
0.340	Ginger Ale
0.339	Milk, nonfat, added Vit A
0.330	Eggplant, boiled, drained, no salt

0.322	Strawberries, raw
0.320	Acerola (West Indian cherry), raw (Missing Sugar and Vitamin Data)
0.310	Beets, canned, drained solids
0.309	Peppers, sweet, red, raw
0.282	Mushrooms, boiled, drained, no salt
0.277	Kale, boiled, drained, no salt
0.271	Spaghetti squash, winter, boiled w/out salt, drained
0.260	Mushrooms, portabella, raw
0.260	Carl's Jr. Italian salad dressing, fat free (Missing Data)
0.250	Lemon juice, raw
0.250	Cauliflower, raw
0.250	Mushrooms, canned, drained solids
0.250	Chicken noodle soup prepared with equal volume water
0.250	Salsa, Campbell Pace, Thick & Chunky (Missing Vitamin Data)
0.241	Tomato sauce, canned
0.230	Cabbage, boiled, drained, no salt
0.230	Basil, fresh
0.228	Spinach, boiled, drained, no salt
0.225	Avg. Leafy Green Vegetables
0.201	Asparagus, raw
0.201	Peppers, sweet, green, raw
0.200	Swiss chard, boiled, drained, no salt
0.181	Tomatoes, raw, red, ripe
0.170	Romaine or cos lettuce
0.164	Radishes, raw
0.161	Zucchini, summer squash, w/ skin, boiled w/out salt, drained
0.150	Cucumber, raw w/ peel
0.140	Iceberg lettuce
0.123	Pickles, cucumber, dill or kosher dill
0.118	Pak-choi, boiled, drained, no salt
0.110	Hot Sauce (ready-to-serve, sauce, pepper or hot)
0.040	Swanson chicken broth, 99% Fat Free
0.008	Chamomile Tea (No O3FA & O6FA Data)
0.008	Black Tea, brewed with tap water
0.007	Coffee, brewed from grounds w/ tap water, no sugar or cream

	(No O3FA Data)

Saturated Fat

Sat Fat, g/SS	Food
0.867	Coconut oil (Missing Trans Fat & O3FA Data)
0.515	Butter, salted (No Trans Fat Data)
0.491	Palm oil (Missing Trans Fat Data)
0.392	Lard (No Trans Fat Data)
0.297	Coconut meat, raw
0.290	Banana chips
0.284	Chocolate-flavored hazelnut spread (No Trans Fat Data)
0.259	Cottonseed (vegetable oil), salad or cooking (Missing Trans Fat Data)
0.259	Nutmeg, ground (Missing O3FA Data)
0.250	Vegetable shortening, household, composite
0.248	Shortening, vegetable, industrial, soy (partially hydrogenated), all purpose
0.221	Dark chocolate candies, 60-69% cacao solids (Missing Vitamin Data)
0.211	Cheddar cheese (No Trans Fat Data)
0.208	Beef sticks, smoked (No Trans Fat Data)
0.204	Margarine, industrial, non-dairy, cottonseed, soy oil (partially hydrogenated), for flaky pastries
0.197	American cheese, pasteurized, w/out disodium phosphate (No Trans Fat Data)
0.193	Cream cheese (No Trans Fat Data)
0.188	Shortening, industrial, soy (partially hydrogenated) for baking & confections (Missing O3FA Data)
0.187	Blue Cheese (No Trans Fat Data)
0.185	Milk chocolate candies (No Trans Fat Data)
0.178	Swiss Cheese (No Trans Fat Data)
0.173	Parmesan cheese, grated (No Trans Fat Data)
0.170	Provolone cheese (No Trans Fat Data)
0.169	Avg. Cheese
0.167	Peanut oil, salad or cooking (No Trans Fat or O3FA Data)
0.156	Soybean oil, salad or cooking (Missing Phytosterol Data)
0.151	Brazil nuts, dried, unblanched
0.149	Pepperoni, pork, beef
0.144	Velveeta cheese, Kraft, pasteurized spread (Missing Data)
0.143	Mayonnaise, Arby's (Missing Vitamin Data)

0.143	Monterey Jack cheese (Missing Data)
0.142	Sesame oil (Missing Trans Fat Data)
0.138	Olive oil (Missing Trans Fat Data)
0.136	Margarine (vegetable oil spread, 70% fat, soybean & partially hydrogenated soybean, stick)
0.133	Bacon (pork), cured, cooked, pan-fried
0.131	Mozzarella cheese, whole milk (No Trans Fat Data)
0.129	Corn oil (vegetable oil), industrial and retail, all purpose salad or cooking
0.125	Hotdog, Oscar Mayer Wiener, beef frank (No Trans Fat Data)
0.120	Macadamia nuts, dry roasted, with salt
0.120	Macadamia nuts, dry roasted, w/out salt
0.119	Mayonnaise, soybean oil, w/ salt (salad dressing)
0.119	Salami, dry or hard, pork (No Trans Fat Data)
0.114	Pork-skins, plain
0.110	Potato chips, plain, salted
0.101	Mozzarella cheese, part skim (No Trans Fat Data)
0.099	Salami, cooked, beef (No Trans Fat Data)
0.099	Spam, Hormel (Missing Data)
0.098	Sunflower oil (vegetable oil) (Missing Trans Fat & Phytosterol Data)
0.096	Grapeseed oil (vegetable oil) (Missing Trans Fat Data)
0.095	Peanut butter, smooth, USDA Commodity
0.095	Sausage, Italian, pork, cooked (No Trans Fat Data)
0.095	Mace, ground (Missing Data)
0.093	Avg. Cased Meat
0.091	Cashews, dry roasted, no salt
0.090	Candy bar, Snickers (King Size)
0.085	Cheetos Crunchy cheese-flavored snacks (No O3, 6FA Data)
0.084	Bay leaf (Missing Data)
0.083	Ricotta cheese, whole milk (No Trans Fat Data)
0.076	T-bone steak, short loin, beef trimmed to 1/8" fat, all grades, broiled
0.075	Ice cream, soft-serve, french vanilla (No Trans Fat Data)
0.074	Avg. Nuts
0.074	Rosemary, dried (Missing Data)
0.074	Canola oil (vegetable oil), low erucic acid rapeseed oil
0.071	Ramen noodle soup, chicken flavor, dry

0.070	Bologna, chicken, pork, beef
0.070	Sage, ground
0.069	Peanuts, dry roasted, no salt, all types
0.069	Popcorn, regular butter flavor, microwave, made w/ partially hydrogenated oil (Missing Fats Data)
0.068	Ice creams, vanilla (No Trans Fat Data)
0.068	Hamburger patty, 80/20 ground chuck beef, broiled
0.065	Sesame sticks, wheat-based, salted
0.063	Pecans, dry roasted, no salt
0.062	Corned beef luncheon meat, beef, cured, canned (No Trans Fat Data)
0.062	Safflower oil (vegetable oil), salad or cooking, linoleic, (over 70%) (No Trans Fat or O3FA Data)
0.062	Walnuts, USDA A259, A257
0.061	Granola bar, soft, uncoated, chocolate chip
0.057	Cheese-flavor puffs or twists, corn-based
0.055	Pistachio nuts, dry roasted, no salt
0.055	Ritz Crackers, Nabisco (Missing Vitamin Data)
0.054	Cloves, ground
0.052	Sunflower Seeds, hulled, dry roased, no salt
0.052	Light mayo (salad dressing)
0.049	Cake, snack cakes, crème-filled, chocolate with frosting
0.045	Poppy seed
0.042	Cap'n Crunch, Quaker
0.042	Banquet chicken pot pie, frozen entrée (Missing Data)
0.042	Slice of pizza, fast food, pizza chain, 14", cheese topping, regular crust (No Trans Fat Data)
0.040	Peanut Butter Cap'n Crunch, Quaker
0.039	Cap'n Crunch with Crunch Berries, Quaker
0.037	Almonds, USDA A256, A264
0.037	Flaxseed
0.037	Egg, whole, cooked, scrambled
0.037	Pumpkin/Squash Seeds, dry roasted, no salt (Missing Vitamin & Se Data)
0.036	Corn chips, extruded, plain
0.036	Popcorn, caramel-coated without peanuts
0.034	Ground turkey, cooked
0.033	Greek style yogurt 150g=2/3 cup (Missing Data)

0.032	Banquest Hearty Ones Salisbury Steak Dinner w/ Gravy, Mashed Potatoes and Corn in Seasoned Sauce, frozen meal(Missing Data)
0.032	Chia seeds, dried (Missing Sugar and Vitamin Data)
0.031	Soybeans (aka soy nuts) mature, dry roasted (Missing Sugar and Vitamin Data)
0.031	Whey protein powder (Low Data)
0.031	Turmeric, ground
0.030	Tortilla chips, plain, white corn
0.030	Chili powder
0.028	Rosemarry, fresh (Missing Data)
0.028	Bologna, lebanon, beef (No O3FA Data)
0.027	Pastrami luncheon meat, beef, cured (No Trans Fat Data)
0.027	Oregano, dried
0.027	Thyme, dried
0.026	Avg. Herbs
0.025	Tortilla chips, plain, yellow corn (Missing Vitamin Data)
0.025	Allspice (Missing Data)
0.023	McDonald's spicy buffalo sauce
0.022	FritoLay Sun Chips, Multi-grain snack, original flavor
0.022	Anchovies, European, canned in oil, drained solids
0.022	Celery seed
0.022	Curry powder
0.021	Avocado, raw, commercial varieties
0.021	Paprika
0.021	Mashed potatoes, home-prepared, whole milk & butter added
0.021	Avg. Spice
0.021	McDonald's French Fries
0.020	Olives, pickled, canned or bottled, green
0.020	Cocoa Krispies, Kellogg's (No O3FA Data)
0.019	Froot Loops, General Mills
0.019	Tarragon, dried (Missing Data)
0.019	Milk, whole, 3.25% milkfat
0.018	Kraft macaroni & cheese dinner, original, unprepared (Missing Data)
0.016	Saffron (Missing Data)
0.015	Wheat dinner rolls
0.015	Oysters, eastern, wild, cooked, moist heat

0.015	Cumin seed
0.015	Mustard seed, yellow
0.015	Fenugreek seed (Missing Vitamin & O3, 6FA Data)
0.014	Swordfish, cooked in dry heat
0.014	Weight Watchers Smart Ones Chicken Enchiladas Suiza, Sour Cream w/ Cheese frozen entrée (Missing Data)
0.014	Cinnamon Toast Crunch cereal, ready-to-eat, General Mills
0.014	Beef, eye of round, separable lean only, trimmed to 0" fat, all grades, roasted [cube steak]
0.013	Soybeans green, boiled, drained, no salt
0.013	Milk, reduced fat, 2%, added Vit A
0.012	Salmon, Atlantic, wild, cooked in dry heat
0.012	Oats
0.012	Popcorn, microwave, 94% fat free
0.012	Pork tenderloin lean, roasted, URMIS 3358
0.011	Hummus, home prepared
0.011	Post Honey Bunches of Oats w/ Almonds (Missing Data)
0.010	Yogurt, regular low-fat, plain, 12 g protein per 8 oz
0.010	Kellogg's Nutri-Grain Cereal Bars, fruit-filled
0.010	Cheerios, General Mills
0.010	Chicken, broilers or fryers, breast, meat only (no skin), roasted
0.010	Black pepper
0.010	Coriander seed (Missing Data)
0.010	Avg. Lean Meat
0.009	Tilapia, cooked in dry heat
0.009	Turkey, stuffing, mashed potatoes w/ gravy, assorted vegetables, frozen, microwaved
0.008	New England clam chowder, Campbell's Select (Missing Data)
0.008	Tuna fish, white, canned in water without salt, drained solids
0.008	Whole wheat bread, prepared from recipe
0.008	Oysters, eastern, wild, raw
0.007	White bread, commercially prepared (inlcudes soft crumbs)
0.007	Whole wheat bread, commecially prepared
0.007	Cardamom (Missing Data)
0.007	Pretzels, soft
0.007	Cottage cheese, 1% milkfat (No Trans Fat Data)
0.007	Avg. Seafood

0.006	Edamame beans, frozen, prepared
0.006	Milk, lowfat, 1%, added Vit A
0.006	Roll, hard, kaiser
0.006	Rice cakes, brown rice, plain
0.006	Popcorn, air-popped
0.006	Lucky Charms, General Mills
0.006	Caraway seed
0.006	Basil, fresh
0.006	Anise seed (Missing Sugar, Vitamin, O3FA data)
0.006	Pretzels, hard, whole-wheat (Missing Sugar Data)
0.006	Honeycomb cereal, Post, Kraft (low data)
0.005	Pretzels, hard, plain, salted
0.005	Wheaties, General Mills
0.005	Ginger, ground
0.005	Marjoram, dried
0.005	Thyme, fresh (Missing Data)
0.005	Fennel seed (Missing Vitamin & O3FA Data)
0.005	Barley (hulled)
0.004	Egg noodles, cooked, enriched
0.004	Whole wheat pita bread
0.004	Bran Flakes, single brand
0.004	Puffed Wheat, Quaker
0.004	Kellogg's Raisin Bran
0.004	Whiting, mixed species, cooked in dry heat
0.004	Flounder (sole), cooked in dry heat
0.004	Red snapper, cooked, dry heat
0.003	Whole wheat flour
0.003	Apple Jacks, Kellogg's
0.003	Honey Smacks, Kellogg's
0.003	Shrimp, mixed species, cooked in moist heat
0.003	Cinnamon
0.003	Oats, unenriched, boiled, w/out salt
0.003	Rye
0.003	Avg. Beans & Lentils
0.002	Chick peas (garbanzo, bengal gram), mature seeds, boiled, no salt
0.002	Tuna fish, light, canned in water without salt, drained solids

0.002	Chicken noodle soup prepared with equal volume water
0.002	Mustard, prepared, yellow
0.002	Bagel, plain, unenriched w/ calcium propionate, onion, poppy, sesame (no cream cheese)
0.002	Brown rice, long-grain, cooked
0.002	White pita bread, enriched
0.002	Matzo crackers, plain
0.002	Corn Flakes, Kellogg's
0.002	Rice Krispies, Kellogg's
0.002	Golden Crisp, Post, Kraft
0.002	Corn Pops, Kellogg's
0.002	Turkey, fryer-roaster, breast meat only, roasted
0.002	Clams, mixed species, cooked in moist heat
0.002	Crayfish, mixed species, farmed, cooked in moist heat
0.002	Basil, dried
0.002	Spearmint, fresh (Missing Data)
0.002	Dill weed, dried (Missing Data)
0.002	Avg. Vegetables
0.002	Corn, sweet, yellow, boiled, drained, no salt
0.002	Millet, cooked
0.002	White flour, white, all-purpose, enriched, bleached
0.001	Banana, raw
0.001	Spaghetti, cooked, enriched w/out added salt, no sauce
0.001	Lobster, northern, cooked in moist heat
0.001	Instant Oatmeal, Quaker, apples & cinnamon prepared w/ boiling water
0.001	Chick peas (garbanzo, bengal gram), mature seeds, canned
0.001	Milk, nonfat, Ca fortified
0.001	Pinto beans, boiled, no salt, mature
0.001	Pomegranate, raw
0.001	Horseradish, prepared
0.001	McDonald's barbeque sauce
0.001	Frosted Flakes, Kellogg's
0.001	Scallops (bay & sea), steamed
0.001	Cilantro, dried (No O3FA Data)
0.001	Parsley, dried (Missing O3FA Data)
0.001	Cantaloupe, raw

0.001	Black beans, mature seeds, canned
0.001	Snap (green string) beans, boiled, drained, no salt
0.001	Kale, boiled, drained, no salt
0.001	Asparagus, raw
0.001	Garlic, raw
0.001	Cherries, sweet, raw
0.001	Papayas, raw
0.001	Broccoli, boiled, drained, no salt
0.001	Mushrooms, shiitake, cooked, no salt
0.001	Peppers, sweet, green, raw
0.001	Grapes, red or green, European type such as Thompson seedless, raw
0.001	Spaghetti squash, winter, boiled w/out salt, drained
0.001	Pickles, cucumber, dill or kosher dill
0.001	Mushrooms, boiled, drained, no salt
0.001	White rice, long-grain, regular, cooked
0.001	Parboiled rice, white, long-grain, enriched, cooked
0.001	Onion, raw
0.001	Potato flour
0.001	Wild rice, cooked
0.001	Mangos, raw
0.001	Raisins, seedless
0.001	Lima beans, immature, boiled, drained, no salt
0.001	White rice, glutinous, cooked
0.001	Kidney beans, red, boiled, no salt, mature seeds
0.001	Spinach, boiled, drained, no salt
0.001	Lentils, mature seeds, boiled, no salt
0.001	Sweet potato, baked in skin, no salt

Unsaturated Fat

Unsaturated fat includes monounsaturated fat and polyunsaturated fat but not trans fat.

Unsaturated Fat, g/SS	Food
0.915	Canola oil (vegetable oil), low erucic acid rapeseed oil
0.891	Safflower oil (vegetable oil), salad or cooking, linoleic, (over 70%) (No Trans Fat or O3FA Data)
0.873	Sunflower oil (vegetable oil) (Missing Trans Fat & Phytosterol Data)
0.858	Grapeseed oil (vegetable oil) (Missing Trans Fat Data)
0.837	Olive oil (Missing Trans Fat Data)
0.822	Corn oil (vegetable oil), industrial and retail, all purpose salad or cooking
0.814	Sesame oil (Missing Trans Fat Data)
0.775	Peanut oil, salad or cooking (No Trans Fat or O3FA Data)
0.760	Shortening, industrial, soy (partially hydrogenated) for baking & confections (Missing O3FA Data)
0.706	Shortening, vegetable, industrial, soy (partially hydrogenated), all purpose
0.696	Cottonseed (vegetable oil), salad or cooking (Missing Trans Fat Data)
0.692	Vegetable shortening, household, composite
0.646	Pecans, dry roasted, no salt
0.643	Mayonnaise, Arby's (Missing Vitamin Data)
0.620	Mayonnaise, soybean oil, w/ salt (salad dressing)
0.608	Macadamia nuts, dry roasted, with salt
0.608	Macadamia nuts, dry roasted, w/out salt
0.563	Lard (No Trans Fat Data)
0.562	Walnuts, USDA A259, A257
0.558	Margarine, industrial, non-dairy, cottonseed, soy oil (partially hydrogenated), for flaky pastries
0.536	Margarine (vegetable oil spread, 70% fat, soybean & partially hydrogenated soybean, stick)
0.490	Avg. Nuts
0.463	Palm oil (Missing Trans Fat Data)
0.452	Brazil nuts, dried, unblanched
0.430	Almonds, USDA A256, A264
0.424	Sunflower Seeds, hulled, dry roased, no salt
0.403	Peanuts, dry roasted, no salt, all types

0.381	Pistachio nuts, dry roasted, no salt
0.351	Cashews, dry roasted, no salt
0.346	Poppy seed
0.321	Peanut butter, smooth, USDA Commodity
0.296	Cheese-flavor puffs or twists, corn-based
0.283	Sesame sticks, wheat-based, salted
0.262	Flaxseed
0.261	Light mayo (salad dressing)
0.254	Chia seeds, dried (Missing Sugar and Vitamin Data)
0.254	Cheetos Crunchy cheese-flavored snacks (No O3, 6FA Data)
0.252	Mustard seed, yellow
0.249	Beef sticks, smoked (No Trans Fat Data)
0.241	Butter, salted (No Trans Fat Data)
0.224	Bacon (pork), cured, cooked, pan-fried
0.220	Potato chips, plain, salted
0.219	Corn chips, extruded, plain
0.206	Pepperoni, pork, beef
0.197	Salami, dry or hard, pork (No Trans Fat Data)
0.195	Celery seed
0.190	Tortilla chips, plain, white corn
0.184	Pork-skins, plain
0.180	FritoLay Sun Chips, Multi-grain snack, original flavor
0.174	Tortilla chips, plain, yellow corn (Missing Vitamin Data)
0.173	Cumin seed
0.172	Ritz Crackers, Nabisco (Missing Vitamin Data)
0.170	Soybeans (aka soy nuts) mature, dry roasted (Missing Sugar and Vitamin Data)
0.168	Spam, Hormel (Missing Data)
0.166	
0.161	Hotdog, Oscar Mayer Wiener, beef frank (No Trans Fat Data)
0.156	Mace, ground (Missing Data)
0.153	Sausage, Italian, pork, cooked (No Trans Fat Data)
0.140	Pumpkin/Squash Seeds, dry roasted, no salt (Missing Vitamin & Se Data)
0.132	Bologna, chicken, pork, beef
0.132	Avg. Cased Meat
0.130	Anise seed (Missing Sugar, Vitamin, O3FA data)

0.126	Olives, pickled, canned or bottled, green
0.126	Dark chocolate candies, 60-69% cacao solids (Missing Vitamin Data)
0.125	McDonald's French Fries
0.116	Avocado, raw, commercial varieties
0.116	Salami, cooked, beef (No Trans Fat Data)
0.116	Fennel seed (Missing Vitamin & O3FA Data)
0.116	McDonald's spicy buffalo sauce
0.111	Chili powder
0.109	Candy bar, Snickers (King Size)
0.106	Avg. Spice
0.104	Caraway seed
0.103	Cheddar cheese (No Trans Fat Data)
0.103	Cake, snack cakes, crème-filled, chocolate with frosting
0.100	Cream cheese (No Trans Fat Data)
0.100	American cheese, pasteurized, w/out disodium phosphate (No Trans Fat Data)
0.096	Parmesan cheese, grated (No Trans Fat Data)
0.095	Paprika
0.092	T-bone steak, short loin, beef trimmed to 1/8" fat, all grades, broiled
0.086	Granola bar, soft, uncoated, chocolate chip
0.086	Blue Cheese (No Trans Fat Data)
0.086	Cloves, ground
0.086	Milk chocolate candies (No Trans Fat Data)
0.085	Avg. Cheese
0.084	Hamburger patty, 80/20 ground chuck beef, broiled
0.083	Swiss Cheese (No Trans Fat Data)
0.082	Curry powder
0.082	Provolone cheese (No Trans Fat Data)
0.081	Ground turkey, cooked
0.076	Coconut oil (Missing Trans Fat & O3FA Data)
0.075	Ramen noodle soup, chicken flavor, dry
0.074	Mozzarella cheese, whole milk (No Trans Fat Data)
0.074	Popcorn, caramel-coated without peanuts
0.070	Soybeans green, boiled, drained, no salt
0.070	Hummus, home prepared

0.069	Egg, whole, cooked, scrambled
0.066	Corned beef luncheon meat, beef, cured, canned (No Trans Fat Data)
0.065	Banquet chicken pot pie, frozen entrée (Missing Data)
0.064	Anchovies, European, canned in oil, drained solids
0.063	Cinnamon Toast Crunch cereal, ready-to-eat, General Mills
0.060	Kellogg's Nutri-Grain Cereal Bars, fruit-filled
0.060	Salmon, Atlantic, wild, cooked in dry heat
0.059	Oregano, dried
0.053	Marjoram, dried
0.053	Rosemary, dried (Missing Data)
0.052	
0.050	Mozzarella cheese, part skim (No Trans Fat Data)
0.050	Popcorn, microwave, 94% fat free
0.050	Banquest Hearty Ones Salisbury Steak Dinner w/ Gravy, Mashed Potatoes and Corn in Seasoned Sauce, frozen meal(Missing Data)
0.049	Fenugreek seed (Missing Vitamin & O3, 6FA Data)
0.048	Peanut Butter Cap'n Crunch, Quaker
0.047	Oats
0.047	Bologna, lebanon, beef (No O3FA Data)
0.042	Wheat dinner rolls
0.042	Tarragon, dried (Missing Data)
0.042	Dill weed, dried (Missing Data)
0.041	Whole wheat bread, prepared from recipe
0.041	Slice of pizza, fast food, pizza chain, 14", cheese topping, regular crust (No Trans Fat Data)
0.040	Ice cream, soft-serve, french vanilla (No Trans Fat Data)
0.040	Ricotta cheese, whole milk (No Trans Fat Data)
0.039	Cheerios, General Mills
0.039	Turmeric, ground
0.039	Bay leaf (Missing Data)
0.039	Avg. Herbs
0.037	Sage, ground
0.037	Parsley, dried (Missing O3FA Data)
0.036	Nutmeg, ground (Missing O3FA Data)
0.036	Mustard, prepared, yellow
0.035	Ice creams, vanilla (No Trans Fat Data)

0.034	Edamame beans, frozen, prepared
0.033	Cocoa Puffs, General Mills
0.032	Swordfish, cooked in dry heat
0.031	Rosemarry, fresh (Missing Data)
0.031	Allspice (Missing Data)
0.030	Popcorn, air-popped
0.028	Roll, hard, kaiser
0.027	Basil, dried
0.025	Banana chips
0.025	Oysters, eastern, wild, cooked, moist heat
0.025	Saffron (Missing Data)
0.025	Cilantro, dried (No O3FA Data)
0.024	Lucky Charms, General Mills
0.023	Turkey, stuffing, mashed potatoes w/ gravy, assorted vegetables, frozen, microwaved
0.023	Pretzels, hard, plain, salted
0.023	Wheaties, General Mills
0.022	Froot Loops, General Mills
0.022	Pastrami luncheon meat, beef, cured (No Trans Fat Data)
0.022	Whole wheat bread, commecially prepared
0.021	White bread, commercially prepared (inlcudes soft crumbs)
0.021	Black pepper
0.020	Pretzels, soft
0.020	Rice cakes, brown rice, plain
0.020	Chicken, broilers or fryers, breast, meat only (no skin), roasted
0.019	Quinoa, cooked
0.019	Beef, eye of round, separable lean only, trimmed to 0" fat, all grades, roasted [cube steak]
0.019	Avg. Seafood
0.019	Tuna fish, white, canned in water without salt, drained solids
0.018	Coconut meat, raw
0.018	Pork tenderloin lean, roasted, URMIS 3358
0.018	Pretzels, hard, whole-wheat (Missing Sugar Data)
0.018	Chick peas (garbanzo, bengal gram), mature seeds, boiled, no salt
0.017	Thyme, dried
0.016	Tilapia, cooked in dry heat

0.016	Honey Smacks, Kellogg's
0.015	Cap'n Crunch, Quaker
0.015	Avg. Lean Meat
0.015	Cap'n Crunch with Crunch Berries, Quaker
0.014	Rye
0.014	Weight Watchers Smart Ones Chicken Enchiladas Suiza, Sour Cream w/ Cheese frozen entrée (Missing Data)
0.014	Whole wheat pita bread
0.014	Puffed Wheat, Quaker
0.014	Barley (hulled)
0.013	Avg. Beans & Lentils
0.013	Bran Flakes, single brand
0.013	Cardamom (Missing Data)
0.013	Oysters, eastern, wild, raw
0.011	Egg noodles, cooked, enriched
0.010	Milk, whole, 3.25% milkfat
0.010	Avg. Vegetables
0.010	Whole wheat flour
0.010	Kellogg's Raisin Bran
0.010	Whiting, mixed species, cooked in dry heat
0.010	Mashed potatoes, home-prepared, whole milk & butter added
0.010	Corn, sweet, yellow, boiled, drained, no salt
0.009	Flounder (sole), cooked in dry heat
0.009	Apple Jacks, Kellogg's
0.009	Red snapper, cooked, dry heat
0.008	Bagel, plain, unenriched w/ calcium propionate, onion, poppy, sesame (no cream cheese)
0.008	McDonald's barbeque sauce
0.008	Clams, mixed species, cooked in moist heat
0.008	Chick peas (garbanzo, bengal gram), mature seeds, canned
0.007	Matzo crackers, plain
0.007	Crayfish, mixed species, farmed, cooked in moist heat
0.007	Ginger, ground
0.007	Millet, cooked
0.007	Chicken noodle soup prepared with equal volume water
0.007	Milk, reduced fat, 2%, added Vit A

0.006	Brown rice, long-grain, cooked
0.006	White pita bread, enriched
0.006	Rice Krispies, Kellogg's
0.006	Shrimp, mixed species, cooked in moist heat
0.006	Scallops (bay & sea), steamed
0.006	Thyme, fresh (Missing Data)
0.006	Cocoa Krispies, Kellogg's (No O3FA Data)
0.005	Tuna fish, light, canned in water without salt, drained solids
0.005	Basil, fresh
0.005	Raspberries, raw
0.005	White flour, white, all-purpose, enriched, bleached
0.004	Yogurt, regular low-fat, plain, 12 g protein per 8 oz
0.004	Spaghetti, cooked, enriched w/out added salt, no sauce
0.004	Horseradish, prepared
0.004	Corn Flakes, Kellogg's
0.004	Spearmint, fresh (Missing Data)
0.004	Corn Pops, Kellogg's
0.004	Cottage cheese, 1% milkfat (No Trans Fat Data)
0.004	Pinto beans, boiled, no salt, mature
0.003	Kidney beans, red, boiled, no salt, mature seeds
0.003	Potato, red, baked, flesh & skin
0.003	Milk, lowfat, 1%, added Vit A
0.003	Turkey, fryer-roaster, breast meat only, roasted
0.003	Cinnamon
0.002	Wild rice, cooked
0.002	Kale, boiled, drained, no salt
0.002	Garlic, raw
0.002	Broccoli, boiled, drained, no salt
0.002	Lobster, northern, cooked in moist heat
0.002	Lentils, mature seeds, boiled, no salt
0.002	Pomegranate, raw
0.002	Romaine or cos lettuce
0.002	Hot Sauce (ready-to-serve, sauce, pepper or hot)
0.002	Acerola (West Indian cherry), raw (Missing Sugar and Vitamin Data)
0.002	Strawberries, raw

0.002	Mushrooms, boiled, drained, no salt
0.002	Mangos, raw
0.002	Lima beans, immature, boiled, drained, no salt
0.002	Peaches, raw
0.002	Black beans, mature seeds, canned
0.002	Ketchup
0.002	Cream of Wheat, instant, prepared with water and salt
0.002	Snap (green string) beans, boiled, drained, no salt
0.002	Peas, frozen, boiled, drained, no salt
0.002	Syrups, maple
0.001	Cherries, sweet, raw
0.001	Avg. Fruit
0.001	Spaghetti squash, winter, boiled w/out salt, drained
0.001	Mushrooms, canned, drained solids
0.001	White rice, long-grain, regular, cooked
0.001	Parboiled rice, white, long-grain, enriched, cooked
0.001	Potato flour
0.001	Grits, corn, white, regular, quick, enriched, cooked with water, with salt
0.001	Tomato sauce, canned
0.001	Raisins, seedless
0.001	Avg. Leafy Green Vegetables
0.001	White rice, glutinous, cooked
0.001	Spinach, boiled, drained, no salt
0.001	Blueberries, raw
0.001	Mushrooms, portabella, raw
0.001	Eggplant, boiled, drained, no salt
0.001	Iceberg lettuce
0.001	Frosted Flakes, Kellogg's
0.001	Salsa, USDA Commodity (Missing Sugar and Vitamin Data)
0.001	Cantaloupe, raw
0.001	Radishes, raw
0.001	Carrots, raw, USDA A099
0.001	Asparagus, raw
0.001	Banana, raw
0.001	Beets, raw

0.001	Papayas, raw
0.001	Mushrooms, shiitake, cooked, no salt
0.001	Beets, canned, drained solids
0.001	Tomatoes, raw, red, ripe
0.001	Peppers, sweet, green, raw
0.001	Peppers, sweet, red, raw
0.001	Potato, baked, flesh & skin, no salt
0.001	Grapes, red or green, European type such as Thompson seedless, raw
0.001	Pickles, cucumber, dill or kosher dill
0.001	Pineapple, raw, all varieties
0.001	White rice, long-grain, pre-cooked or instant, prepared (Missing O3FA Data)
0.001	Pak-choi, boiled, drained, no salt
0.001	Pineapple, canned, juice pack, drained
0.001	Sweet potato, baked in skin, no salt

Trans Fat

Trans Fat, g/SS	Food
0.429	Shortening, industrial, soy (partially hydrogenated) for baking & confections (Missing O3FA Data)
0.342	Shortening, vegetable, industrial, soy (partially hydrogenated), all purpose
0.247	Margarine, industrial, non-dairy, cottonseed, soy oil (partially hydrogenated), for flaky pastries
0.148	Margarine (vegetable oil spread, 70% fat, soybean & partially hydrogenated soybean, stick)
0.132	Vegetable shortening, household, composite
0.095	Popcorn, regular butter flavor, microwave, made w/ partially hydrogenated oil (Missing Fats Data)
0.016	Pepperoni, pork, beef
0.012	Hamburger patty, 80/20 ground chuck beef, broiled
0.011	Ritz Crackers, Nabisco (Missing Vitamin Data)
0.010	Honey Smacks, Kellogg's
0.009	Popcorn, microwave, 94% fat free
0.009	Avg. Cased Meat
0.008	Whole wheat bread, commecially prepared
0.008	Cheese-flavor puffs or twists, corn-based
0.007	Corn chips, extruded, plain
0.006	Egg, whole, cooked, scrambled
0.005	Banquest Hearty Ones Salisbury Steak Dinner w/ Gravy, Mashed Potatoes and Corn in Seasoned Sauce, frozen meal(Missing Data)
0.004	Candy bar, Snickers (King Size)
0.004	Canola oil (vegetable oil), low erucic acid rapeseed oil
0.003	Corn oil (vegetable oil), industrial and retail, all purpose salad or cooking
0.003	Mayonnaise, soybean oil, w/ salt (salad dressing)
0.002	Bologna, chicken, pork, beef
0.002	McDonald's French Fries
0.002	Banquet chicken pot pie, frozen entrée (Missing Data)
0.001	Mashed potatoes, home-prepared, whole milk & butter added
0.001	Weight Watchers Smart Ones Chicken Enchiladas Suiza, Sour Cream w/ Cheese frozen entrée (Missing Data)
0.001	Tortilla chips, plain, white corn
0.001	FritoLay Sun Chips, Multi-grain snack, original flavor

0.001	Light mayo (salad dressing)
0.001	McDonald's spicy buffalo sauce
0.001	Cinnamon Toast Crunch cereal, ready-to-eat, General Mills
0.001	Cap'n Crunch with Crunch Berries, Quaker
0.001	Corn Pops, Kellogg's
0.001	Tortilla chips, plain, yellow corn (Missing Vitamin Data)
0.001	Dark chocolate candies, 60-69% cacao solids (Missing Vitamin Data)

Cholesterol

Cholesterol, mg/SS	Food
3.520	Egg, whole, cooked, scrambled
2.150	Butter, salted (No Trans Fat Data)
1.950	Shrimp, mixed species, cooked in moist heat
1.370	Crayfish, mixed species, farmed, cooked in moist heat
1.330	Beef sticks, smoked (No Trans Fat Data)
1.130	Bacon (pork), cured, cooked, pan-fried
1.099	Cream cheese (No Trans Fat Data)
1.094	Whey protein powder (Low Data)
1.071	Monterey Jack cheese (Missing Data)
1.053	Cheddar cheese (No Trans Fat Data)
1.050	Oysters, eastern, wild, cooked, moist heat
1.050	Pepperoni, pork, beef
1.020	Ground turkey, cooked
0.951	Lard (No Trans Fat Data)
0.950	Pork-skins, plain
0.940	American cheese, pasteurized, w/out disodium phosphate (No Trans Fat Data)
0.917	Swiss Cheese (No Trans Fat Data)
0.910	Ice cream, soft-serve, french vanilla (No Trans Fat Data)
0.910	Hamburger patty, 80/20 ground chuck beef, broiled
0.887	
0.880	Parmesan cheese, grated (No Trans Fat Data)
0.860	Corned beef luncheon meat, beef, cured, canned (No Trans Fat Data)
0.850	Chicken, broilers or fryers, breast, meat only (no skin), roasted
0.850	Anchovies, European, canned in oil, drained solids
0.847	Avg. Cheese
0.840	Whiting, mixed species, cooked in dry heat
0.830	Turkey, fryer-roaster, breast meat only, roasted
0.830	Bologna, chicken, pork, beef
0.800	Velveeta cheese, Kraft, pasteurized spread (Missing Data)
0.788	Salami, dry or hard, pork (No Trans Fat Data)
0.786	Mozzarella cheese, whole milk (No Trans Fat Data)
0.752	Avg. Cased Meat

0.750	Blue Cheese (No Trans Fat Data)
0.749	Avg. Seafood
0.740	Avg. Lean Meat
0.730	Pork tenderloin lean, roasted, URMIS 3358
0.717	Lobster, northern, cooked in moist heat
0.710	Salami, cooked, beef (No Trans Fat Data)
0.710	Mayonnaise, Arby's (Missing Vitamin Data)
0.708	Salmon, Atlantic, wild, cooked in dry heat
0.700	Spam, Hormel (Missing Data)
0.690	Provolone cheese (No Trans Fat Data)
0.680	Pastrami luncheon meat, beef, cured (No Trans Fat Data)
0.677	Flounder (sole), cooked in dry heat
0.670	Clams, mixed species, cooked in moist heat
0.640	Mozzarella cheese, part skim (No Trans Fat Data)
0.620	T-bone steak, short loin, beef trimmed to 1/8" fat, all grades, broiled
0.570	Tilapia, cooked in dry heat
0.560	Hotdog, Oscar Mayer Wiener, beef frank (No Trans Fat Data)
0.550	Beef, eye of round, separable lean only, trimmed to 0" fat, all grades, roasted [cube steak]
0.550	Bologna, lebanon, beef (No O3FA Data)
0.540	Sausage, Italian, pork, cooked (No Trans Fat Data)
0.530	Scallops (bay & sea), steamed
0.528	Oysters, eastern, wild, raw
0.522	
0.510	Ricotta cheese, whole milk (No Trans Fat Data)
0.500	Swordfish, cooked in dry heat
0.471	Red snapper, cooked, dry heat
0.440	Ice creams, vanilla (No Trans Fat Data)
0.419	Tuna fish, white, canned in water without salt, drained solids
0.382	Mayonnaise, soybean oil, w/ salt (salad dressing)
0.350	Light mayo (salad dressing)
0.303	Tuna fish, light, canned in water without salt, drained solids
0.288	Egg noodles, cooked, enriched
0.232	Milk chocolate candies (No Trans Fat Data)
0.230	Cheetos Crunchy cheese-flavored snacks (No O3, 6FA Data)

0.214	Slice of pizza, fast food, pizza chain, 14", cheese topping, regular crust (No Trans Fat Data)
0.152	Banquet chicken pot pie, frozen entrée (Missing Data)
0.141	Banquest Hearty Ones Salisbury Steak Dinner w/ Gravy, Mashed Potatoes and Corn in Seasoned Sauce, frozen meal(Missing Data)
0.140	Turkey, stuffing, mashed potatoes w/ gravy, assorted vegetables, frozen, microwaved
0.140	Kraft macaroni & cheese dinner, original, unprepared (Missing Data)
0.133	Greek style yogurt 150g=2/3 cup (Missing Data)
0.133	Candy bar, Snickers (King Size)
0.129	Weight Watchers Smart Ones Chicken Enchiladas Suiza, Sour Cream w/ Cheese frozen entrée (Missing Data)
0.110	Mashed potatoes, home-prepared, whole milk & butter added
0.100	Milk, whole, 3.25% milkfat
0.082	Milk, reduced fat, 2%, added Vit A
0.070	Cheese-flavor puffs or twists, corn-based
0.063	Dark chocolate candies, 60-69% cacao solids (Missing Vitamin Data)
0.061	Yogurt, regular low-fat, plain, 12 g protein per 8 oz
0.050	Popcorn, caramel-coated without peanuts
0.049	Milk, lowfat, 1%, added Vit A
0.048	Chicken noodle soup prepared with equal volume water
0.041	New England clam chowder, Campbell's Select (Missing Data)
0.040	Popcorn, regular butter flavor, microwave, made w/ partially hydrogenated oil (Missing Fats Data)
0.040	Cottage cheese, 1% milkfat (No Trans Fat Data)
0.028	Pretzels, soft
0.020	Milk, nonfat, Ca fortified
0.020	Milk, nonfat, added Vit A

Total Omega-3 Fatty Acids

TO3FA mg/SS	Food
228.130	Flaxseed
175.520	Chia seeds, dried (Missing Sugar and Vitamin Data)
91.381	Canola oil (vegetable oil), low erucic acid rapeseed oil
90.795	Walnuts, USDA A259, A257
67.890	Soybean oil, salad or cooking (Missing Phytosterol Data)
47.027	Mayonnaise, soybean oil, w/ salt (salad dressing)
42.790	Cloves, ground
41.800	Oregano, dried
32.300	Marjoram, dried
29.550	Tarragon, dried (Missing Data)
26.800	Mustard seed, yellow
25.857	Salmon, Atlantic, wild, cooked in dry heat
21.678	Avg. Herbs
21.130	Anchovies, European, canned in oil, drained solids
20.750	Margarine (vegetable oil spread, 70% fat, soybean & partially hydrogenated soybean, stick)
19.180	Light mayo (salad dressing)
18.829	Vegetable shortening, household, composite
15.090	Basil, dried
14.430	Soybeans (aka soy nuts) mature, dry roasted (Missing Sugar and Vitamin Data)
13.450	Oysters, eastern, wild, cooked, moist heat
12.480	Saffron (Missing Data)
12.300	Sage, ground
12.186	Avg. Nuts
11.970	Ritz Crackers, Nabisco (Missing Vitamin Data)
11.610	Corn oil (vegetable oil), industrial and retail, all purpose salad or cooking
10.760	Rosemary, dried (Missing Data)
10.566	Swordfish, cooked in dry heat
10.500	Bay leaf (Missing Data)
10.000	Lard (No Trans Fat Data)
9.940	Pecans, dry roasted, no salt
9.700	Sesame sticks, wheat-based, salted
9.620	McDonald's spicy buffalo sauce

9.512	Tuna fish, white, canned in water without salt, drained solids
9.271	Avg. Spice
9.000	Paprika
7.860	Margarine, industrial, non-dairy, cottonseed, soy oil (partially hydrogenated), for flaky pastries
7.611	Olive oil (Missing Trans Fat Data)
7.339	Avg. Seafood
7.310	Chili powder
6.900	Thyme, dried
6.722	Oysters, eastern, wild, raw
5.983	Soybeans green, boiled, drained, no salt
5.630	Flounder (sole), cooked in dry heat
5.480	Whiting, mixed species, cooked in dry heat
4.910	Tortilla chips, plain, yellow corn (Missing Vitamin Data)
4.880	Mustard, prepared, yellow
4.820	Turmeric, ground
4.470	Thyme, fresh (Missing Data)
4.400	Sausage, Italian, pork, cooked (No Trans Fat Data)
4.290	Curry powder
4.140	Rosemarry, fresh (Missing Data)
4.000	Popcorn, caramel-coated without peanuts
3.960	Scallops (bay & sea), steamed
3.960	Clams, mixed species, cooked in moist heat
3.830	American cheese, pasteurized, w/out disodium phosphate (No Trans Fat Data)
3.800	Beef sticks, smoked (No Trans Fat Data)
3.770	Salami, cooked, beef (No Trans Fat Data)
3.723	Mozzarella cheese, whole milk (No Trans Fat Data)
3.652	Cheddar cheese (No Trans Fat Data)
3.630	Tortilla chips, plain, white corn
3.613	Edamame beans, frozen, prepared
3.547	McDonald's French Fries
3.523	Swiss Cheese (No Trans Fat Data)
3.470	Shrimp, mixed species, cooked in moist heat
3.429	Red snapper, cooked, dry heat
3.380	Spearmint, fresh (Missing Data)
3.170	Whole wheat bread, prepared from recipe

3.160	Basil, fresh
3.150	Butter, salted (No Trans Fat Data)
3.030	Cheese-flavor puffs or twists, corn-based
3.000	Sesame oil (Missing Trans Fat Data)
2.796	Salami, dry or hard, pork (No Trans Fat Data)
2.788	Tuna fish, light, canned in water without salt, drained solids
2.763	Avg. Cheese
2.750	Provolone cheese (No Trans Fat Data)
2.730	Poppy seed
2.653	
2.640	Blue Cheese (No Trans Fat Data)
2.618	Pistachio nuts, dry roasted, no salt
2.600	Pork-skins, plain
2.400	Tilapia, cooked in dry heat
2.390	Hotdog, Oscar Mayer Wiener, beef frank (No Trans Fat Data)
2.390	Avg. Cased Meat
2.212	Corn chips, extruded, plain
2.100	Corned beef luncheon meat, beef, cured, canned (No Trans Fat Data)
2.100	Spam, Hormel (Missing Data)
2.092	Shortening, vegetable, industrial, soy (partially hydrogenated), all purpose
2.000	T-bone steak, short loin, beef trimmed to 1/8" fat, all grades, broiled
2.000	Ground turkey, cooked
2.000	Celery seed
2.000	Palm oil (Missing Trans Fat Data)
2.000	Cottonseed (vegetable oil), salad or cooking (Missing Trans Fat Data)
1.962	Macadamia nuts, dry roasted, with salt
1.962	Macadamia nuts, dry roasted, w/out salt
1.922	Sunflower oil (vegetable oil) (Missing Trans Fat & Phytosterol Data)
1.900	Parmesan cheese, grated (No Trans Fat Data)
1.899	Potato chips, plain, salted
1.890	Bacon (pork), cured, cooked, pan-fried
1.870	Pepperoni, pork, beef
1.840	Crayfish, mixed species, farmed, cooked in moist heat
1.800	Ice cream, soft-serve, french vanilla (No Trans Fat Data)
1.780	Ice creams, vanilla (No Trans Fat Data)

1.760	Cumin seed
1.730	Cake, snack cakes, crème-filled, chocolate with frosting
1.728	Cream cheese (No Trans Fat Data)
1.689	Slice of pizza, fast food, pizza chain, 14", cheese topping, regular crust (No Trans Fat Data)
1.680	Bologna, chicken, pork, beef
1.678	Kidney beans, red, boiled, no salt, mature seeds
1.613	Cashews, dry roasted, no salt
1.600	Black pepper
1.568	Rye
1.540	Cinnamon Toast Crunch cereal, ready-to-eat, General Mills
1.500	Caraway seed
1.439	Avg. Beans & Lentils
1.390	White bread, commercially prepared (inlcudes soft crumbs)
1.370	Mozzarella cheese, part skim (No Trans Fat Data)
1.368	Pinto beans, boiled, no salt, mature
1.260	Raspberries, raw
1.220	Milk chocolate candies (No Trans Fat Data)
1.200	Cardamom (Missing Data)
1.189	Broccoli, boiled, drained, no salt
1.160	Egg, whole, cooked, scrambled
1.130	Romaine or cos lettuce
1.120	Ricotta cheese, whole milk (No Trans Fat Data)
1.109	Oats
1.100	Avocado, raw, commercial varieties
1.098	Barley (hulled)
1.031	Kale, boiled, drained, no salt
1.021	Turkey, stuffing, mashed potatoes w/ gravy, assorted vegetables, frozen, microwaved
1.010	Wheaties, General Mills
1.000	Grapeseed oil (vegetable oil) (Missing Trans Fat Data)
0.970	Roll, hard, kaiser
0.951	Wild rice, cooked
0.930	FritoLay Sun Chips, Multi-grain snack, original flavor
0.922	Spinach, boiled, drained, no salt
0.920	Olives, pickled, canned or bottled, green
0.890	Cheerios, General Mills

0.888	Snap (green string) beans, boiled, drained, no salt
0.880	Dark chocolate candies, 60-69% cacao solids (Missing Vitamin Data)
0.862	Lobster, northern, cooked in moist heat
0.830	
0.812	Ginger, ground
0.800	Mace, ground (Missing Data)
0.781	Spaghetti squash, winter, boiled w/out salt, drained
0.770	Pumpkin/Squash Seeds, dry roasted, no salt (Missing Vitamin & Se Data)
0.760	McDonald's barbeque sauce
0.750	Milk, whole, 3.25% milkfat
0.740	Pretzels, hard, plain, salted
0.740	Hummus, home prepared
0.700	Bran Flakes, single brand
0.700	Chicken, broilers or fryers, breast, meat only (no skin), roasted
0.700	Allspice (Missing Data)
0.693	Avg. Leafy Green Vegetables
0.690	Sunflower Seeds, hulled, dry roased, no salt
0.650	Strawberries, raw
0.600	Popcorn, air-popped
0.600	Granola bar, soft, uncoated, chocolate chip
0.590	Puffed Wheat, Quaker
0.580	Blueberries, raw
0.580	Wheat dinner rolls
0.580	Froot Loops, General Mills
0.571	Black beans, mature seeds, canned
0.560	Kellogg's Nutri-Grain Cereal Bars, fruit-filled
0.560	Kellogg's Raisin Bran
0.560	Lucky Charms, General Mills
0.550	Popcorn, microwave, 94% fat free
0.550	Ramen noodle soup, chicken flavor, dry
0.530	Horseradish, prepared
0.520	Iceberg lettuce
0.520	Whole wheat pita bread
0.512	Peanut butter, smooth, USDA Commodity
0.500	Lima beans, immature, boiled, drained, no salt

0.480	Hamburger patty, 80/20 ground chuck beef, broiled
0.480	Candy bar, Snickers (King Size)
0.460	Cantaloupe, raw
0.440	Acerola (West Indian cherry), raw (Missing Sugar and Vitamin Data)
0.430	Chick peas (garbanzo, bengal gram), mature seeds, boiled, no salt
0.420	Honey Smacks, Kellogg's
0.410	Pak-choi, boiled, drained, no salt
0.400	Pretzels, hard, whole-wheat (Missing Sugar Data)
0.380	Whole wheat flour
0.370	Mangos, raw
0.370	Lentils, mature seeds, boiled, no salt
0.370	Cauliflower, raw
0.360	Bagel, plain, unenriched w/ calcium propionate, onion, poppy, sesame (no cream cheese)
0.350	Potato flour
0.340	Peanut Butter Cap'n Crunch, Quaker
0.326	Avg. Fruit
0.320	Matzo crackers, plain
0.320	Pickles, cucumber, dill or kosher dill
0.310	Radishes, raw
0.285	Avg. Lean Meat
0.280	Egg noodles, cooked, enriched
0.280	Millet, cooked
0.270	Cap'n Crunch with Crunch Berries, Quaker
0.270	Banana, raw
0.260	Cherries, sweet, raw
0.260	Mashed potatoes, home-prepared, whole milk & butter added
0.250	Papayas, raw
0.250	Whole wheat bread, commecially prepared
0.250	Peppers, sweet, red, raw
0.240	Butternut squash, winter, baked w/out salt, sugar or butter
0.240	Spaghetti, cooked, enriched w/out added salt, no sauce
0.240	White pita bread, enriched
0.240	Cap'n Crunch, Quaker
0.240	Peas, frozen, boiled, drained, no salt
0.239	Avg. Vegetables

0.230	Cranberry juice cocktail, bottled
0.220	White flour, white, all-purpose, enriched, bleached
0.200	Corn Flakes, Kellogg's
0.200	Turkey, fryer-roaster, breast meat only, roasted
0.200	Garlic, raw
0.190	Chick peas (garbanzo, bengal gram), mature seeds, canned
0.180	Apple Jacks, Kellogg's
0.180	Oats, unenriched, boiled, w/out salt
0.180	Corn, sweet, yellow, boiled, drained, no salt
0.180	Chicken noodle soup prepared with equal volume water
0.180	Brazil nuts, dried, unblanched
0.170	Pineapple, raw, all varieties
0.170	Parboiled rice, white, long-grain, enriched, cooked
0.170	Pineapple, canned, juice pack, drained
0.170	Rice Krispies, Kellogg's
0.150	Eggplant, boiled, drained, no salt
0.140	Cabbage, boiled, drained, no salt
0.140	Brown rice, long-grain, cooked
0.140	Cream of Wheat, instant, prepared with water and salt
0.130	Yogurt, regular low-fat, plain, 12 g protein per 8 oz
0.130	Instant Oatmeal, Quaker, apples & cinnamon prepared w/ boiling water
0.130	Potato, baked, flesh & skin, no salt
0.130	Zucchini, summer squash, w/ skin, boiled w/out salt, drained
0.130	Pork tenderloin lean, roasted, URMIS 3358
0.130	White rice, long-grain, regular, cooked
0.110	Beef, eye of round, separable lean only, trimmed to 0" fat, all grades, roasted [cube steak]
0.110	Pastrami luncheon meat, beef, cured (No Trans Fat Data)
0.110	Cinnamon
0.110	Grapes, red or green, European type such as Thompson seedless, raw
0.100	Asparagus, raw
0.100	Banana chips
0.100	Rice cakes, brown rice, plain
0.100	Potato, red, baked, flesh & skin
0.100	Potato, Russet, baked, flesh & skin
0.090	Apple, raw, with skin A343

0.090	Cottage cheese, 1% milkfat (No Trans Fat Data)
0.080	Milk, reduced fat, 2%, added Vit A
0.080	Peppers, sweet, green, raw
0.072	Orange, raw, all commercial varieties
0.070	Raisins, seedless
0.070	Apple Juice, canned or bottled, unsweetened
0.061	Pretzels, soft
0.060	Almonds, USDA A256, A264
0.060	Corn Pops, Kellogg's
0.060	Frosted Flakes, Kellogg's
0.050	Grape Juice, canned or bottled, unsweetened
0.050	Cucumber, raw w/ peel
0.050	Beets, raw
0.040	Syrups, maple
0.040	Milk, lowfat, 1%, added Vit A
0.040	Beets, canned, drained solids
0.040	Onion, raw
0.040	Sweet potato, baked in skin, no salt
0.040	Ketchup
0.040	Soy sauce, low sodium (soy & wheat)
0.040	Rice noodles, cooked (Missing Sugar & Unsaturated Fat Data)
0.030	Mushrooms, shiitake, cooked, no salt
0.030	Swiss chard, boiled, drained, no salt
0.030	Tomato sauce, canned
0.030	Tomatoes, raw, red, ripe
0.030	Peanuts, dry roasted, no salt, all types
0.030	Black Tea, brewed with tap water
0.030	White rice, glutinous, cooked
0.020	Carrots, raw, USDA A099
0.020	Peaches, raw
0.020	Soy sauce (soy & wheat)
0.020	Milk, nonfat, Ca fortified
0.020	Grits, corn, white, regular, quick, enriched, cooked with water, with salt
0.010	Mushrooms, boiled, drained, no salt
0.010	Mushrooms, canned, drained solids

0.010	Milk, nonfat, added Vit A
0.010	Mushrooms, portabella, raw
0.010	Hot Sauce (ready-to-serve, sauce, pepper or hot)
0.010	Salsa, USDA Commodity (Missing Sugar and Vitamin Data)

Total Omega-6 Fatty Acids

TO6FA mg/SS	Food
746.151	Safflower oil (vegetable oil), salad or cooking, linoleic, (over 70%) (No Trans Fat or O3FA Data)
695.908	Grapeseed oil (vegetable oil) (Missing Trans Fat Data)
535.096	Corn oil (vegetable oil), industrial and retail, all purpose salad or cooking
515.028	Cottonseed (vegetable oil), salad or cooking (Missing Trans Fat Data)
504.225	Soybean oil, salad or cooking (Missing Phytosterol Data)
413.037	Sesame oil (Missing Trans Fat Data)
380.915	Walnuts, USDA A259, A257
376.782	Mayonnaise, soybean oil, w/ salt (salad dressing)
327.852	Sunflower Seeds, hulled, dry roasted, no salt
317.115	Peanut oil, salad or cooking (No Trans Fat or O3FA Data)
282.910	Poppy seed
262.171	Vegetable shortening, household, composite
205.639	Brazil nuts, dried, unblanched
195.780	Pecans, dry roasted, no salt
186.450	Canola oil (vegetable oil), low erucic acid rapeseed oil
181.720	Margarine (vegetable oil spread, 70% fat, soybean & partially hydrogenated soybean, stick)
180.850	Cheese-flavor puffs or twists, corn-based
164.390	Sesame sticks, wheat-based, salted
160.370	Light mayo (salad dressing)
157.904	Avg. Nuts
156.911	Peanuts, dry roasted, no salt, all types
137.899	Corn chips, extruded, plain
136.358	Pistachio nuts, dry roasted, no salt
120.650	Almonds, USDA A256, A264
119.802	Potato chips, plain, salted
118.500	Tortilla chips, plain, white corn
112.814	Peanut butter, smooth, USDA Commodity
107.645	Soybeans (aka soy nuts) mature, dry roasted (Missing Sugar and Vitamin Data)
101.990	Lard (No Trans Fat Data)
97.630	Olive oil (Missing Trans Fat Data)
97.010	Ritz Crackers, Nabisco (Missing Vitamin Data)

91.000	Palm oil (Missing Trans Fat Data)
87.590	Pumpkin/Squash Seeds, dry roasted, no salt (Missing Vitamin & Se Data)
85.913	Shortening, vegetable, industrial, soy (partially hydrogenated), all purpose
84.790	Margarine, industrial, non-dairy, cottonseed, soy oil (partially hydrogenated), for flaky pastries
76.606	Cashews, dry roasted, no salt
74.210	Paprika
74.160	McDonald's spicy buffalo sauce
67.260	Chili powder
65.930	Tortilla chips, plain, yellow corn (Missing Vitamin Data)
63.560	FritoLay Sun Chips, Multi-grain snack, original flavor
59.110	Flaxseed
57.850	Chia seeds, dried (Missing Sugar and Vitamin Data)
50.000	Shortening, industrial, soy (partially hydrogenated) for baking & confections (Missing O3FA Data)
44.657	Soybeans green, boiled, drained, no salt
43.110	Mace, ground (Missing Data)
42.402	McDonald's French Fries
41.010	Bacon (pork), cured, cooked, pan-fried
40.700	Popcorn, caramel-coated without peanuts
40.290	Beef sticks, smoked (No Trans Fat Data)
36.055	Sunflower oil (vegetable oil) (Missing Trans Fat & Phytosterol Data)
35.200	Celery seed
33.500	Pork-skins, plain
32.699	Salami, dry or hard, pork (No Trans Fat Data)
32.180	Bologna, chicken, pork, beef
31.500	Anise seed (Missing Sugar, Vitamin, O3FA data)
31.220	Caraway seed
31.030	Cumin seed
30.815	Avg. Spice
29.655	Candy bar, Snickers (King Size)
29.100	Ground turkey, cooked
29.050	Cinnamon Toast Crunch cereal, ready-to-eat, General Mills
28.950	Pepperoni, pork, beef
28.400	Sausage, Italian, pork, cooked (No Trans Fat Data)
27.400	Spam, Hormel (Missing Data)

27.282	Butter, salted (No Trans Fat Data)
26.210	Whole wheat bread, prepared from recipe
25.900	Mustard seed, yellow
25.860	Cloves, ground
24.990	Popcorn, air-popped
24.237	Oats
22.900	Allspice (Missing Data)
21.610	Popcorn, microwave, 94% fat free
21.260	Peanut Butter Cap'n Crunch, Quaker
21.200	Curry powder
20.346	Hummus, home prepared
19.160	Egg, whole, cooked, scrambled
18.800	Cheerios, General Mills
17.995	Coconut oil (Missing Trans Fat & O3FA Data)
17.962	Avg. Cased Meat
17.942	Edamame beans, frozen, prepared
17.500	Coriander seed (Missing Data)
16.940	Turmeric, ground
16.900	Fennel seed (Missing Vitamin & O3FA Data)
16.896	Avocado, raw, commercial varieties
16.490	Cake, snack cakes, crème-filled, chocolate with frosting
16.210	Roll, hard, kaiser
15.160	Granola bar, soft, uncoated, chocolate chip
14.194	Slice of pizza, fast food, pizza chain, 14", cheese topping, regular crust (No Trans Fat Data)
13.320	Ramen noodle soup, chicken flavor, dry
13.030	Macadamia nuts, dry roasted, with salt
13.030	Macadamia nuts, dry roasted, w/out salt
12.400	Bay leaf (Missing Data)
12.185	Milk chocolate candies (No Trans Fat Data)
12.160	White bread, commercially prepared (inlcudes soft crumbs)
12.150	Olives, pickled, canned or bottled, green
11.750	Marjoram, dried
11.600	Rosemary, dried (Missing Data)
11.430	Froot Loops, General Mills
11.268	Dark chocolate candies, 60-69% cacao solids (Missing Vitamin Data)

11.250	Lucky Charms, General Mills
11.128	Chick peas (garbanzo, bengal gram), mature seeds, boiled, no salt
10.650	Wheaties, General Mills
10.500	Oregano, dried
10.490	Wheat dinner rolls
10.319	Cream cheese (No Trans Fat Data)
10.080	Puffed Wheat, Quaker
10.010	Whole wheat pita bread
9.989	Barley (hulled)
9.980	Pretzels, hard, plain, salted
9.700	Rice cakes, brown rice, plain
9.700	Black pepper
9.652	Turkey, stuffing, mashed potatoes w/ gravy, assorted vegetables, frozen, microwaved
9.580	Rye
9.520	Bran Flakes, single brand
9.510	Hotdog, Oscar Mayer Wiener, beef frank (No Trans Fat Data)
9.430	Parmesan cheese, grated (No Trans Fat Data)
8.923	Pretzels, soft
8.500	Kellogg's Nutri-Grain Cereal Bars, fruit-filled
8.460	Honey Smacks, Kellogg's
7.900	Pretzels, hard, whole-wheat (Missing Sugar Data)
7.828	Avg. Herbs
7.762	Avg. Beans & Lentils
7.730	Cap'n Crunch with Crunch Berries, Quaker
7.660	Cap'n Crunch, Quaker
7.540	Saffron (Missing Data)
7.420	Tarragon, dried (Missing Data)
7.383	Whole wheat flour
6.740	Kellogg's Raisin Bran
6.603	Bagel, plain, unenriched w/ calcium propionate, onion, poppy, sesame (no cream cheese)
6.600	Salami, cooked, beef (No Trans Fat Data)
6.590	Basil, dried
6.205	Swiss Cheese (No Trans Fat Data)
6.200	Banana chips
6.084	Avg. Cheese

6.070	American cheese, pasteurized, w/out disodium phosphate (No Trans Fat Data)
5.900	Chicken, broilers or fryers, breast, meat only (no skin), roasted
5.860	Corn, sweet, yellow, boiled, drained, no salt
5.773	Cheddar cheese (No Trans Fat Data)
5.740	Whole wheat bread, commecially prepared
5.700	Matzo crackers, plain
5.410	Oats, unenriched, boiled, w/out salt
5.360	Blue Cheese (No Trans Fat Data)
5.300	Sage, ground
5.219	Egg noodles, cooked, enriched
5.110	White pita bread, enriched
5.000	Thyme, dried
4.939	Provolone cheese (No Trans Fat Data)
4.908	Chick peas (garbanzo, bengal gram), mature seeds, canned
4.799	Millet, cooked
4.790	Apple Jacks, Kellogg's
4.599	T-bone steak, short loin, beef trimmed to 1/8" fat, all grades, broiled
4.580	Parsley, dried (Missing O3FA Data)
4.550	Mustard, prepared, yellow
4.470	Rosemarry, fresh (Missing Data)
4.240	Pork tenderloin lean, roasted, URMIS 3358
4.230	McDonald's barbeque sauce
4.200	Corned beef luncheon meat, beef, cured, canned (No Trans Fat Data)
4.110	Hamburger patty, 80/20 ground chuck beef, broiled
3.929	Mozzarella cheese, whole milk (No Trans Fat Data)
3.912	White flour, white, all-purpose, enriched, bleached
3.660	Coconut meat, raw
3.620	Anchovies, European, canned in oil, drained solids
3.500	Nutmeg, ground (Missing O3FA Data)
3.350	Mozzarella cheese, part skim (No Trans Fat Data)
3.280	Cilantro, dried (No O3FA Data)
3.158	Avg. Lean Meat
3.100	Cardamom (Missing Data)
3.092	Brown rice, long-grain, cooked
3.000	Corn Flakes, Kellogg's

3.000	Tilapia, cooked in dry heat
2.950	Spaghetti, cooked, enriched w/out added salt, no sauce
2.860	Ginger, ground
2.850	Horseradish, prepared
2.800	Ice cream, soft-serve, french vanilla (No Trans Fat Data)
2.780	Rice Krispies, Kellogg's
2.752	Instant Oatmeal, Quaker, apples & cinnamon prepared w/ boiling water
2.750	Ice creams, vanilla (No Trans Fat Data)
2.730	Ricotta cheese, whole milk (No Trans Fat Data)
2.488	Raspberries, raw
2.460	Bologna, lebanon, beef (No O3FA Data)
2.419	Chicken noodle soup prepared with equal volume water
2.300	Cocoa Krispies, Kellogg's (No O3FA Data)
2.287	Garlic, raw
2.201	Salmon, Atlantic, wild, cooked in dry heat
1.950	Hot Sauce (ready-to-serve, sauce, pepper or hot)
1.940	Corn Pops, Kellogg's
1.897	Mushrooms, boiled, drained, no salt
1.813	Avg. Vegetables
1.560	Crayfish, mixed species, farmed, cooked in moist heat
1.369	Lentils, mature seeds, boiled, no salt
1.329	Mashed potatoes, home-prepared, whole milk & butter added
1.300	Turkey, fryer-roaster, breast meat only, roasted
1.208	Ketchup
1.201	Milk, whole, 3.25% milkfat
1.199	Cream of Wheat, instant, prepared with water and salt
1.190	Beef, eye of round, separable lean only, trimmed to 0" fat, all grades, roasted [cube steak]
1.189	Wild rice, cooked
1.170	Oysters, eastern, wild, cooked, moist heat
1.160	Mushrooms, canned, drained solids
1.160	Pastrami luncheon meat, beef, cured (No Trans Fat Data)
1.148	Carrots, raw, USDA A099
1.119	Potato flour
1.068	Kidney beans, red, boiled, no salt, mature seeds
1.060	Salsa, USDA Commodity (Missing Sugar and Vitamin Data)

1.051	Peas, frozen, boiled, drained, no salt
1.041	Lima beans, immature, boiled, drained, no salt
1.000	Syrups, maple
0.982	Pinto beans, boiled, no salt, mature
0.960	Frosted Flakes, Kellogg's
0.956	Avg. Seafood
0.901	Strawberries, raw
0.880	Blueberries, raw
0.850	Thyme, fresh (Missing Data)
0.840	Peaches, raw
0.810	Grits, corn, white, regular, quick, enriched, cooked with water, with salt
0.799	Tomatoes, raw, red, ripe
0.792	Kale, boiled, drained, no salt
0.790	Pomegranate, raw
0.780	Eggplant, boiled, drained, no salt
0.750	Mushrooms, portabella, raw
0.741	Parboiled rice, white, long-grain, enriched, cooked
0.730	Basil, fresh
0.690	Tomato sauce, canned
0.679	Black beans, mature seeds, canned
0.661	White rice, glutinous, cooked
0.620	White rice, long-grain, regular, cooked
0.619	Milk, reduced fat, 2%, added Vit A
0.600	Sweet potato, baked in skin, no salt
0.600	Avg. Fruit
0.581	Oysters, eastern, wild, raw
0.560	Snap (green string) beans, boiled, drained, no salt
0.557	Beets, raw
0.550	Tuna fish, white, canned in water without salt, drained solids
0.540	Peppers, sweet, green, raw
0.540	Spearmint, fresh (Missing Data)
0.511	Broccoli, boiled, drained, no salt
0.470	Romaine or cos lettuce
0.470	Spaghetti squash, winter, boiled w/out salt, drained
0.460	Banana, raw

0.460	Acerola (West Indian cherry), raw (Missing Sugar and Vitamin Data)
0.450	Peppers, sweet, red, raw
0.449	Beets, canned, drained solids
0.440	Cinnamon
0.431	Potato, baked, flesh & skin, no salt
0.430	Apple, raw, with skin A343
0.400	Asparagus, raw
0.370	Avg. Leafy Green Vegetables
0.370	Grapes, red or green, European type such as Thompson seedless, raw
0.370	Swordfish, cooked in dry heat
0.350	Cranberry juice cocktail, bottled
0.350	Cantaloupe, raw
0.330	Apple Juice, canned or bottled, unsweetened
0.320	Potato, red, baked, flesh & skin
0.320	Potato, Russet, baked, flesh & skin
0.320	Clams, mixed species, cooked in moist heat
0.320	Soy sauce, low sodium (soy & wheat)
0.310	Mushrooms, shiitake, cooked, no salt
0.310	Yogurt, regular low-fat, plain, 12 g protein per 8 oz
0.310	Pak-choi, boiled, drained, no salt
0.300	Milk, lowfat, 1%, added Vit A
0.290	Raisins, seedless
0.280	Cucumber, raw w/ peel
0.270	Cherries, sweet, raw
0.250	Red snapper, cooked, dry heat
0.250	Corn starch (Missing O3FA Data)
0.250	Swiss chard, boiled, drained, no salt
0.240	Pickles, cucumber, dill or kosher dill
0.230	Pineapple, raw, all varieties
0.230	Pineapple, canned, juice pack, drained
0.220	Cottage cheese, 1% milkfat (No Trans Fat Data)
0.210	Iceberg lettuce
0.210	Shrimp, mixed species, cooked in moist heat
0.200	Whiting, mixed species, cooked in dry heat
0.190	Rice noodles, cooked (Missing Sugar & Unsaturated Fat Data)
0.184	Orange, raw, all commercial varieties

0.170	White rice, long-grain, pre-cooked or instant, prepared (Missing O3FA Data)
0.170	Spinach, boiled, drained, no salt
0.170	Grape Juice, canned or bottled, unsweetened
0.170	Radishes, raw
0.160	Soy sauce (soy & wheat)
0.140	Flounder (sole), cooked in dry heat
0.140	Mangos, raw
0.140	Butternut squash, winter, baked w/out salt, sugar or butter
0.130	Onion, raw
0.110	Cauliflower, raw
0.090	Cabbage, boiled, drained, no salt
0.090	Tuna fish, light, canned in water without salt, drained solids
0.080	Zucchini, summer squash, w/ skin, boiled w/out salt, drained
0.070	Scallops (bay & sea), steamed
0.060	Papayas, raw
0.050	Lobster, northern, cooked in moist heat
0.050	Milk, nonfat, Ca fortified
0.020	Milk, nonfat, added Vit A
0.010	Black Tea, brewed with tap water
0.009	Coffee, brewed from grounds w/ tap water, no sugar or cream (No O3FA Data)

Ratio of Total Omega-3 Fatty Acids to Total Omega-6 Fatty Acids

TO3FA/ TO6FA Ratio	Food
56.571	Scallops (bay & sea), steamed
40.169	Flounder (sole), cooked in dry heat
31.081	Tuna fish, light, canned in water without salt, drained solids
28.571	Swordfish, cooked in dry heat
27.400	Whiting, mixed species, cooked in dry heat
17.294	Tuna fish, white, canned in water without salt, drained solids
17.123	Lobster, northern, cooked in moist heat
16.524	Shrimp, mixed species, cooked in moist heat
13.718	Red snapper, cooked, dry heat
12.375	Clams, mixed species, cooked in moist heat
11.746	Salmon, Atlantic, wild, cooked in dry heat
11.576	Oysters, eastern, wild, raw
11.496	Oysters, eastern, wild, cooked, moist heat
7.675	Avg. Seafood
6.259	Spearmint, fresh (Missing Data)
5.837	Anchovies, European, canned in oil, drained solids
5.425	Spinach, boiled, drained, no salt
5.259	Thyme, fresh (Missing Data)
4.329	Basil, fresh
4.167	Papayas, raw
3.982	Tarragon, dried (Missing Data)
3.981	Oregano, dried
3.859	Flaxseed
3.364	Cauliflower, raw
3.034	Chia seeds, dried (Missing Sugar and Vitamin Data)
2.958	Black Tea, brewed with tap water
2.769	Avg. Herbs
2.749	Marjoram, dried
2.645	Mangos, raw
2.476	Iceberg lettuce
2.404	Romaine or cos lettuce
2.329	Broccoli, boiled, drained, no salt

2.321	Sage, ground
2.290	Basil, dried
1.872	Avg. Leafy Green Vegetables
1.827	Radishes, raw
1.714	Butternut squash, winter, baked w/out salt, sugar or butter
1.662	Spaghetti squash, winter, boiled w/out salt, drained
1.655	Saffron (Missing Data)
1.655	Cloves, ground
1.625	Zucchini, summer squash, w/ skin, boiled w/out salt, drained
1.586	Snap (green string) beans, boiled, drained, no salt
1.571	Kidney beans, red, boiled, no salt, mature seeds
1.556	Cabbage, boiled, drained, no salt
1.393	Pinto beans, boiled, no salt, mature
1.380	Thyme, dried
1.333	Pickles, cucumber, dill or kosher dill
1.323	Pak-choi, boiled, drained, no salt
1.314	Cantaloupe, raw
1.301	Kale, boiled, drained, no salt
1.179	Crayfish, mixed species, farmed, cooked in moist heat
1.072	Mustard, prepared, yellow
1.035	Mustard seed, yellow
0.962	Cherries, sweet, raw
0.957	Acerola (West Indian cherry), raw (Missing Sugar and Vitamin Data)
0.948	Mozzarella cheese, whole milk (No Trans Fat Data)
0.928	Rosemary, dried (Missing Data)
0.926	Rosemarry, fresh (Missing Data)
0.847	Bay leaf (Missing Data)
0.840	Black beans, mature seeds, canned
0.800	Wild rice, cooked
0.800	Tilapia, cooked in dry heat
0.740	Pineapple, canned, juice pack, drained
0.739	Pineapple, raw, all varieties
0.721	Strawberries, raw
0.659	Blueberries, raw
0.657	Cranberry juice cocktail, bottled
0.647	Ice creams, vanilla (No Trans Fat Data)

0.643	Ice cream, soft-serve, french vanilla (No Trans Fat Data)
0.633	Cheddar cheese (No Trans Fat Data)
0.631	American cheese, pasteurized, w/out disodium phosphate (No Trans Fat Data)
0.625	Milk, whole, 3.25% milkfat
0.586	Banana, raw
0.571	Salami, cooked, beef (No Trans Fat Data)
0.568	Swiss Cheese (No Trans Fat Data)
0.557	Provolone cheese (No Trans Fat Data)
0.555	Peppers, sweet, red, raw
0.544	Avg. Fruit
0.510	Milk, nonfat, added Vit A
0.507	Raspberries, raw
0.500	Corned beef luncheon meat, beef, cured, canned (No Trans Fat Data)
0.493	Blue Cheese (No Trans Fat Data)
0.490	Canola oil (vegetable oil), low erucic acid rapeseed oil
0.480	Lima beans, immature, boiled, drained, no salt
0.454	Avg. Cheese
0.435	T-bone steak, short loin, beef trimmed to 1/8" fat, all grades, broiled
0.420	Yogurt, regular low-fat, plain, 12 g protein per 8 oz
0.410	Ricotta cheese, whole milk (No Trans Fat Data)
0.409	Mozzarella cheese, part skim (No Trans Fat Data)
0.408	Cottage cheese, 1% milkfat (No Trans Fat Data)
0.395	Milk, nonfat, Ca fortified
0.390	Orange, raw, all commercial varieties
0.387	Cardamom (Missing Data)
0.313	Potato flour
0.312	Potato, red, baked, flesh & skin
0.312	Potato, Russet, baked, flesh & skin
0.308	Onion, raw
0.302	Potato, baked, flesh & skin, no salt
0.301	Avg. Spice
0.297	Grapes, red or green, European type such as Thompson seedless, raw
0.295	Grape Juice, canned or bottled, unsweetened
0.285	Turmeric, ground
0.284	Ginger, ground

0.270	Lentils, mature seeds, boiled, no salt
0.251	Hotdog, Oscar Mayer Wiener, beef frank (No Trans Fat Data)
0.250	Asparagus, raw
0.250	Cinnamon
0.243	Raisins, seedless
0.238	Walnuts, USDA A259, A257
0.230	Parboiled rice, white, long-grain, enriched, cooked
0.228	Peas, frozen, boiled, drained, no salt
0.212	Apple Juice, canned or bottled, unsweetened
0.210	Apple, raw, with skin A343
0.210	Rice noodles, cooked (Missing Sugar & Unsaturated Fat Data)
0.209	White rice, long-grain, regular, cooked
0.202	Curry powder
0.201	Parmesan cheese, grated (No Trans Fat Data)
0.201	Edamame beans, frozen, prepared
0.196	Mashed potatoes, home-prepared, whole milk & butter added
0.192	Eggplant, boiled, drained, no salt
0.186	Horseradish, prepared
0.185	Avg. Beans & Lentils
0.180	McDonald's barbeque sauce
0.179	Cucumber, raw w/ peel
0.168	Cream cheese (No Trans Fat Data)
0.165	Black pepper
0.164	Rye
0.155	Sausage, Italian, pork, cooked (No Trans Fat Data)
0.154	Turkey, fryer-roaster, breast meat only, roasted
0.151	Macadamia nuts, dry roasted, with salt
0.151	Macadamia nuts, dry roasted, w/out salt
0.148	Peppers, sweet, green, raw
0.135	Soybean oil, salad or cooking (Missing Phytosterol Data)
0.134	Soybeans (aka soy nuts) mature, dry roasted (Missing Sugar and Vitamin Data)
0.134	Soybeans green, boiled, drained, no salt
0.134	Milk, lowfat, 1%, added Vit A
0.133	Avg. Cased Meat
0.132	Avg. Vegetables

0.130	McDonald's spicy buffalo sauce
0.129	Milk, reduced fat, 2%, added Vit A
0.125	Soy sauce (soy & wheat)
0.125	Soy sauce, low sodium (soy & wheat)
0.125	Mayonnaise, soybean oil, w/ salt (salad dressing)
0.123	Ritz Crackers, Nabisco (Missing Vitamin Data)
0.121	Swiss chard, boiled, drained, no salt
0.121	Paprika
0.121	Whole wheat bread, prepared from recipe
0.120	Light mayo (salad dressing)
0.119	Slice of pizza, fast food, pizza chain, 14", cheese topping, regular crust (No Trans Fat Data)
0.119	Chicken, broilers or fryers, breast, meat only (no skin), roasted
0.117	Hamburger patty, 80/20 ground chuck beef, broiled
0.117	Cream of Wheat, instant, prepared with water and salt
0.115	Butter, salted (No Trans Fat Data)
0.114	White bread, commercially prepared (inlcudes soft crumbs)
0.114	Margarine (vegetable oil spread, 70% fat, soybean & partially hydrogenated soybean, stick)
0.110	Barley (hulled)
0.109	Chili powder
0.106	Turkey, stuffing, mashed potatoes w/ gravy, assorted vegetables, frozen, microwaved
0.105	Cake, snack cakes, crème-filled, chocolate with frosting
0.100	Milk chocolate candies (No Trans Fat Data)
0.098	Popcorn, caramel-coated without peanuts
0.098	Lard (No Trans Fat Data)
0.098	Mushrooms, shiitake, cooked, no salt
0.095	Wheaties, General Mills
0.095	Pastrami luncheon meat, beef, cured (No Trans Fat Data)
0.094	Beef sticks, smoked (No Trans Fat Data)
0.093	Margarine, industrial, non-dairy, cottonseed, soy oil (partially hydrogenated), for flaky pastries
0.092	Beef, eye of round, separable lean only, trimmed to 0" fat, all grades, roasted [cube steak]
0.090	Avg. Lean Meat
0.090	Beets, raw
0.089	Beets, canned, drained solids

0.087	Garlic, raw
0.086	Salami, dry or hard, pork (No Trans Fat Data)
0.084	McDonald's French Fries
0.083	Kellogg's Raisin Bran
0.081	Spaghetti, cooked, enriched w/out added salt, no sauce
0.078	Dark chocolate candies, 60-69% cacao solids (Missing Vitamin Data)
0.078	Olive oil (Missing Trans Fat Data)
0.078	Pork-skins, plain
0.077	Avg. Nuts
0.077	Spam, Hormel (Missing Data)
0.076	Olives, pickled, canned or bottled, green
0.074	Tortilla chips, plain, yellow corn (Missing Vitamin Data)
0.074	Chicken noodle soup prepared with equal volume water
0.074	Pretzels, hard, plain, salted
0.074	Bran Flakes, single brand
0.072	Vegetable shortening, household, composite
0.069	Ground turkey, cooked
0.067	Sweet potato, baked in skin, no salt
0.067	Corn Flakes, Kellogg's
0.066	Kellogg's Nutri-Grain Cereal Bars, fruit-filled
0.065	Avocado, raw, commercial varieties
0.065	Pepperoni, pork, beef
0.063	Frosted Flakes, Kellogg's
0.061	Rice Krispies, Kellogg's
0.061	Egg, whole, cooked, scrambled
0.060	Roll, hard, kaiser
0.059	Sesame sticks, wheat-based, salted
0.059	Puffed Wheat, Quaker
0.058	Millet, cooked
0.057	Celery seed
0.057	Cumin seed
0.056	White flour, white, all-purpose, enriched, bleached
0.056	Matzo crackers, plain
0.055	Wheat dinner rolls
0.055	Bagel, plain, unenriched w/ calcium propionate, onion, poppy, sesame (no cream cheese)

Ratio of Total Omega-3 Fatty Acids to Total Omega-6 Fatty Acids

0.054	Egg noodles, cooked, enriched
0.053	Sunflower oil (vegetable oil) (Missing Trans Fat & Phytosterol Data)
0.053	Cinnamon Toast Crunch cereal, ready-to-eat, General Mills
0.052	Bologna, chicken, pork, beef
0.052	Whole wheat pita bread
0.051	Whole wheat flour
0.051	Pecans, dry roasted, no salt
0.051	Froot Loops, General Mills
0.051	Pretzels, hard, whole-wheat (Missing Sugar Data)
0.050	Lucky Charms, General Mills
0.050	Honey Smacks, Kellogg's
0.048	Caraway seed
0.047	Cheerios, General Mills
0.047	Instant Oatmeal, Quaker, apples & cinnamon prepared w/ boiling water
0.047	White pita bread, enriched
0.046	Bacon (pork), cured, cooked, pan-fried
0.046	Oats
0.045	Brown rice, long-grain, cooked
0.045	White rice, glutinous, cooked
0.044	Tomato sauce, canned
0.044	Whole wheat bread, commecially prepared
0.041	Ramen noodle soup, chicken flavor, dry
0.040	Syrups, maple
0.040	Granola bar, soft, uncoated, chocolate chip
0.039	Chick peas (garbanzo, bengal gram), mature seeds, canned
0.039	Chick peas (garbanzo, bengal gram), mature seeds, boiled, no salt
0.038	Tomatoes, raw, red, ripe
0.038	Apple Jacks, Kellogg's
0.036	Hummus, home prepared
0.035	Cap'n Crunch with Crunch Berries, Quaker
0.033	Oats, unenriched, boiled, w/out salt
0.033	Ketchup
0.031	Cap'n Crunch, Quaker
0.031	Corn Pops, Kellogg's
0.031	Corn, sweet, yellow, boiled, drained, no salt

0.031	Pork tenderloin lean, roasted, URMIS 3358
0.031	Tortilla chips, plain, white corn
0.031	Allspice (Missing Data)
0.025	Popcorn, microwave, 94% fat free
0.024	Grits, corn, white, regular, quick, enriched, cooked with water, with salt
0.024	Shortening, vegetable, industrial, soy (partially hydrogenated), all purpose
0.024	Popcorn, air-popped
0.024	Peaches, raw
0.022	Palm oil (Missing Trans Fat Data)
0.022	Corn oil (vegetable oil), industrial and retail, all purpose salad or cooking
0.021	Cashews, dry roasted, no salt
0.019	Pistachio nuts, dry roasted, no salt
0.019	Mace, ground (Missing Data)
0.018	Carrots, raw, USDA A099
0.017	Cheese-flavor puffs or twists, corn-based
0.016	Candy bar, Snickers (King Size)
0.016	Banana chips
0.016	Corn chips, extruded, plain
0.016	Peanut Butter Cap'n Crunch, Quaker
0.016	Potato chips, plain, salted
0.015	FritoLay Sun Chips, Multi-grain snack, original flavor
0.013	Mushrooms, portabella, raw
0.010	Rice cakes, brown rice, plain
0.010	Poppy seed
0.009	Salsa, USDA Commodity (Missing Sugar and Vitamin Data)
0.009	Mushrooms, canned, drained solids
0.009	Pumpkin/Squash Seeds, dry roasted, no salt (Missing Vitamin & Se Data)
0.007	Sesame oil (Missing Trans Fat Data)
0.007	Pretzels, soft
0.005	Mushrooms, boiled, drained, no salt
0.005	Hot Sauce (ready-to-serve, sauce, pepper or hot)
0.005	Peanut butter, smooth, USDA Commodity
0.004	Cottonseed (vegetable oil), salad or cooking (Missing Trans Fat Data)
0.002	Sunflower Seeds, hulled, dry roasted, no salt

Ratio of Total Omega-3 Fatty Acids to Total Omega-6 Fatty Acids

0.001	Grapeseed oil (vegetable oil) (Missing Trans Fat Data)
0.001	Brazil nuts, dried, unblanched

Fiber

Fiber, g/SS	Food
0.530	Cinnamon
0.428	Oregano, dried
0.426	Rosemary, dried (Missing Data)
0.420	Coriander seed (Missing Data)
0.403	Sage, ground
0.400	Avg. Herbs
0.400	Basil, dried
0.400	Marjoram, dried
0.400	Fennel seed (Missing Vitamin & O3FA Data)
0.380	Caraway seed
0.377	Chia seeds, dried (Missing Sugar and Vitamin Data)
0.374	Paprika
0.370	Thyme, dried
0.340	Chili powder
0.340	Cloves, ground
0.330	Curry powder
0.304	Parsley, dried (Missing O3FA Data)
0.286	Avg. Spice
0.280	Cardamom (Missing Data)
0.273	Flaxseed
0.265	Black pepper
0.260	Bay leaf (Missing Data)
0.250	Fenugreek seed (Missing Vitamin & O3, 6FA Data)
0.220	Allspice (Missing Data)
0.211	Turmeric, ground
0.210	Nutmeg, ground (Missing O3FA Data)
0.200	Mace, ground (Missing Data)
0.195	Poppy seed
0.176	Bran Flakes, single brand
0.173	Barley (hulled)
0.150	Mustard seed, yellow
0.150	Anise seed (Missing Sugar, Vitamin, O3FA data)
0.146	Rye

0.145	Popcorn, air-popped
0.141	Rosemarry, fresh (Missing Data)
0.140	Thyme, fresh (Missing Data)
0.140	Dill weed, dried (Missing Data)
0.136	Popcorn, microwave, 94% fat free
0.122	Almonds, USDA A256, A264
0.122	Whole wheat flour
0.120	Celery seed
0.111	Kellogg's Raisin Bran
0.111	Sunflower Seeds, hulled, dry roased, no salt
0.110	Cumin seed
0.106	Oats
0.103	Pistachio nuts, dry roasted, no salt
0.101	Cheerios, General Mills
0.100	Wheaties, General Mills
0.100	Cilantro, dried (No O3FA Data)
0.099	Popcorn, regular butter flavor, microwave, made w/ partially hydrogenated oil (Missing Fats Data)
0.094	Pecans, dry roasted, no salt
0.094	Puffed Wheat, Quaker
0.090	Pinto beans, boiled, no salt, mature
0.090	Coconut meat, raw
0.085	Avg. Nuts
0.081	Soybeans (aka soy nuts) mature, dry roasted (Missing Sugar and Vitamin Data)
0.080	Dark chocolate candies, 60-69% cacao solids (Missing Vitamin Data)
0.080	Macadamia nuts, dry roasted, with salt
0.080	Macadamia nuts, dry roasted, w/out salt
0.080	Peanuts, dry roasted, no salt, all types
0.079	Lentils, mature seeds, boiled, no salt
0.077	Banana chips
0.077	Pretzels, hard, whole-wheat (Missing Sugar Data)
0.076	Chick peas (garbanzo, bengal gram), mature seeds, boiled, no salt
0.075	Brazil nuts, dried, unblanched
0.074	Kidney beans, red, boiled, no salt, mature seeds
0.074	Whole wheat pita bread

0.074	Tarragon, dried (Missing Data)
0.069	Black beans, mature seeds, canned
0.068	Whole wheat bread, commecially prepared
0.068	FritoLay Sun Chips, Multi-grain snack, original flavor
0.068	Spearmint, fresh (Missing Data)
0.067	Avocado, raw, commercial varieties
0.067	Walnuts, USDA A259, A257
0.065	Raspberries, raw
0.062	Avg. Beans & Lentils
0.060	Whole wheat bread, prepared from recipe
0.059	Potato flour
0.058	Soybeans green, boiled, drained, no salt
0.057	Peanut butter, smooth, USDA Commodity
0.055	Peas, frozen, boiled, drained, no salt
0.054	Chocolate-flavored hazelnut spread (No Trans Fat Data)
0.053	Corn chips, extruded, plain
0.053	Tortilla chips, plain, white corn
0.053	Lima beans, immature, boiled, drained, no salt
0.052	Edamame beans, frozen, prepared
0.052	Popcorn, caramel-coated without peanuts
0.050	Cocoa Puffs, General Mills
0.050	Agave nectar (Missing Data)
0.050	Post Honey Bunches of Oats w/ Almonds (Missing Data)
0.047	Lucky Charms, General Mills
0.047	Tortilla chips, plain, yellow corn (Missing Vitamin Data)
0.044	Chick peas (garbanzo, bengal gram), mature seeds, canned
0.044	Potato chips, plain, salted
0.042	Rice cakes, brown rice, plain
0.042	McDonald's French Fries
0.040	Pomegranate, raw
0.040	Ginger, ground
0.040	Hummus, home prepared
0.039	Saffron (Missing Data)
0.038	Wheat dinner rolls
0.038	Granola bar, soft, uncoated, chocolate chip
0.038	Cinnamon Toast Crunch cereal, ready-to-eat, General Mills

0.037	Honey Smacks, Kellogg's
0.037	Raisins, seedless
0.034	Milk chocolate candies (No Trans Fat Data)
0.033	Sweet potato, baked in skin, no salt
0.033	Olives, pickled, canned or bottled, green
0.033	Horseradish, prepared
0.033	Mustard, prepared, yellow
0.033	Broccoli, boiled, drained, no salt
0.032	Snap (green string) beans, boiled, drained, no salt
0.032	Cake, snack cakes, crème-filled, chocolate with frosting
0.031	Froot Loops, General Mills
0.031	Salsa, Campbell Pace, Thick & Chunky (Missing Vitamin Data)
0.030	Matzo crackers, plain
0.030	Pretzels, hard, plain, salted
0.030	Cashews, dry roasted, no salt
0.028	Carrots, raw, USDA A099
0.028	Quinoa, cooked
0.028	Corn, sweet, yellow, boiled, drained, no salt
0.028	Sesame sticks, wheat-based, salted
0.028	Cheetos Crunchy cheese-flavored snacks (No O3, 6FA Data)
0.028	Beets, raw
0.027	White flour, white, all-purpose, enriched, bleached
0.027	Peanut Butter Cap'n Crunch, Quaker
0.026	Banana, raw
0.025	Eggplant, boiled, drained, no salt
0.025	Cauliflower, raw
0.025	Corn Flakes, Kellogg's
0.025	Cap'n Crunch, Quaker
0.025	Cap'n Crunch with Crunch Berries, Quaker
0.025	Honeycomb cereal, Post, Kraft (low data)
0.024	Orange, raw, all commercial varieties
0.024	Apple, raw, with skin A343
0.024	Blueberries, raw
0.024	White bread, commercially prepared (inlcudes soft crumbs)
0.024	Ramen noodle soup, chicken flavor, dry
0.024	Spinach, boiled, drained, no salt

0.024	Mushrooms, canned, drained solids
0.023	Avg. Fruit
0.023	Potato, Russet, baked, flesh & skin
0.023	Candy bar, Snickers (King Size)
0.023	Roll, hard, kaiser
0.023	Ritz Crackers, Nabisco (Missing Vitamin Data)
0.023	Bagel, plain, unenriched w/ calcium propionate, onion, poppy, sesame (no cream cheese)
0.022	Avg. Vegetables
0.022	Potato, baked, flesh & skin, no salt
0.022	White pita bread, enriched
0.022	Mushrooms, boiled, drained, no salt
0.021	Garlic, raw
0.021	Swiss chard, boiled, drained, no salt
0.021	Avg. Leafy Green Vegetables
0.021	Cherries, sweet, raw
0.021	Romaine or cos lettuce
0.021	Kellogg's Nutri-Grain Cereal Bars, fruit-filled
0.021	Kraft macaroni & cheese dinner, original, unprepared (Missing Data)
0.021	Banquest Hearty Ones Salisbury Steak Dinner w/ Gravy, Mashed Potatoes and Corn in Seasoned Sauce, frozen meal(Missing Data)
0.021	Asparagus, raw
0.021	Peppers, sweet, red, raw
0.021	Mushrooms, shiitake, cooked, no salt
0.020	Kale, boiled, drained, no salt
0.020	Strawberries, raw
0.019	Cabbage, boiled, drained, no salt
0.019	Cheese-flavor puffs or twists, corn-based
0.019	Cocoa Krispies, Kellogg's (No O3FA Data)
0.018	Wild rice, cooked
0.018	Mangos, raw
0.018	Instant Oatmeal, Quaker, apples & cinnamon prepared w/ boiling water
0.018	Potato, red, baked, flesh & skin
0.018	Beets, canned, drained solids
0.018	Frosted Flakes, Kellogg's
0.018	Brown rice, long-grain, cooked

0.018	Papayas, raw
0.018	Spaghetti, cooked, enriched w/out added salt, no sauce
0.017	Slice of pizza, fast food, pizza chain, 14", cheese topping, regular crust (No Trans Fat Data)
0.017	Banquet chicken pot pie, frozen entrée (Missing Data)
0.017	Oats, unenriched, boiled, w/out salt
0.017	Onion, raw
0.017	Pretzels, soft
0.017	Peppers, sweet, green, raw
0.016	Radishes, raw
0.016	Apple Jacks, Kellogg's
0.016	Basil, fresh
0.015	Tomato sauce, canned
0.015	Mushrooms, portabella, raw
0.015	McDonald's spicy buffalo sauce
0.015	Peaches, raw
0.015	Mashed potatoes, home-prepared, whole milk & butter added
0.014	Spaghetti squash, winter, boiled w/out salt, drained
0.014	Butternut squash, winter, baked w/out salt, sugar or butter
0.014	Salsa, USDA Commodity (Missing Sugar and Vitamin Data)
0.014	Pineapple, raw, all varieties
0.014	Zucchini, summer squash, w/ skin, boiled w/out salt, drained
0.013	Pineapple, canned, juice pack, drained
0.013	Millet, cooked
0.013	McDonald's barbeque sauce
0.013	Turkey, stuffing, mashed potatoes w/ gravy, assorted vegetables, frozen, microwaved
0.013	Weight Watchers Smart Ones Chicken Enchiladas Suiza, Sour Cream w/ Cheese frozen entrée (Missing Data)
0.012	Tomatoes, raw, red, ripe
0.012	Iceberg lettuce
0.012	Egg noodles, cooked, enriched
0.011	Pickles, cucumber, dill or kosher dill
0.010	Rice noodles, cooked (Missing Sugar & Unsaturated Fat Data)
0.010	Pak-choi, boiled, drained, no salt
0.010	Acerola (West Indian cherry), raw (Missing Sugar and Vitamin Data)
0.010	White rice, glutinous, cooked

0.009	Corn starch (Missing O3FA Data)
0.009	Grapes, red or green, European type such as Thompson seedless, raw
0.009	Parboiled rice, white, long-grain, enriched, cooked
0.009	Cantaloupe, raw
0.008	New England clam chowder, Campbell's Select (Missing Data)
0.008	Rice Krispies, Kellogg's
0.008	Corn Pops, Kellogg's
0.008	Soy sauce (soy & wheat)
0.008	Soy sauce, low sodium (soy & wheat)
0.007	Ice creams, vanilla (No Trans Fat Data)
0.007	Ice cream, soft-serve, french vanilla (No Trans Fat Data)
0.006	White rice, long-grain, pre-cooked or instant, prepared (Missing O3FA Data)
0.006	Cream of Wheat, instant, prepared with water and salt
0.005	Cucumber, raw w/ peel
0.004	Lemon juice, raw
0.004	White rice, long-grain, regular, cooked
0.003	Apricot jam and preserves
0.003	Honey
0.003	Ketchup
0.003	Grits, corn, white, regular, quick, enriched, cooked with water, with salt
0.002	Chicken noodle soup prepared with equal volume water
0.002	Grape Juice, canned or bottled, unsweetened
0.002	Apple Juice, canned or bottled, unsweetened
0.001	Teriyaki sauce, ready-to-serve
0.001	Sausage, Italian, pork, cooked (No Trans Fat Data)

Sugar

Sugar, g/SS	Food
0.999	Sugars, granulated (sucrose)
0.968	Brown sugars
0.820	Honey
0.710	Agave nectar (Missing Data)
0.643	Strawberry Jam, Hardee's condiment (Missing Data)
0.596	Syrups, maple
0.592	Raisins, seedless
0.560	Honey Smacks, Kellogg's
0.540	Chocolate-flavored hazelnut spread (No Trans Fat Data)
0.539	Golden Crisp, Post, Kraft
0.532	Popcorn, caramel-coated without peanuts
0.515	Milk chocolate candies (No Trans Fat Data)
0.504	Candy bar, Snickers (King Size)
0.479	Corn Pops, Kellogg's
0.467	Cocoa Puffs, General Mills
0.450	Froot Loops, General Mills
0.447	Cap'n Crunch with Crunch Berries, Quaker
0.438	Cap'n Crunch, Quaker
0.434	Apricot jam and preserves
0.416	Apple Jacks, Kellogg's
0.399	Lucky Charms, General Mills
0.387	Frosted Flakes, Kellogg's
0.383	Honeycomb cereal, Post, Kraft (low data)
0.378	Cake, snack cakes, crème-filled, chocolate with frosting
0.367	Dark chocolate candies, 60-69% cacao solids (Missing Vitamin Data)
0.353	Banana chips
0.351	Kellogg's Nutri-Grain Cereal Bars, fruit-filled
0.343	McDonald's barbeque sauce
0.340	Cocoa Krispies, Kellogg's (No O3FA Data)
0.332	Cinnamon Toast Crunch cereal, ready-to-eat, General Mills
0.331	Peanut Butter Cap'n Crunch, Quaker
0.299	Kellogg's Raisin Bran
0.289	Granola bar, soft, uncoated, chocolate chip

0.280	Nutmeg, ground (Missing O3FA Data)
0.264	High-fructose corn syrup
0.228	Ketchup
0.212	Ice creams, vanilla (No Trans Fat Data)
0.212	Ice cream, soft-serve, french vanilla (No Trans Fat Data)
0.210	Post Honey Bunches of Oats w/ Almonds (Missing Data)
0.189	Bran Flakes, single brand
0.155	Grapes, red or green, European type such as Thompson seedless, raw
0.148	Mangos, raw
0.143	Pineapple, canned, juice pack, drained
0.142	Grape Juice, canned or bottled, unsweetened
0.141	Teriyaki sauce, ready-to-serve
0.137	Pomegranate, raw
0.133	Wheaties, General Mills
0.130	Weight Watchers Smart Ones Chicken Enchiladas Suiza, Sour Cream w/ Cheese frozen entrée (Missing Data)
0.128	Cherries, sweet, raw
0.122	Banana, raw
0.120	Coca Cola Classic
0.119	Cranberry juice cocktail, bottled
0.114	Pepsi (Missing Data)
0.105	Corn Flakes, Kellogg's
0.104	Apple, raw, with skin A343
0.103	Paprika
0.100	Avg. Fruit
0.100	Blueberries, raw
0.100	Kraft macaroni & cheese dinner, original, unprepared (Missing Data)
0.099	Pineapple, raw, all varieties
0.096	Apple Juice, canned or bottled, unsweetened
0.096	Orange, raw, all commercial varieties
0.095	Rice Krispies, Kellogg's
0.090	Sprite
0.087	Ginger Ale
0.084	Peaches, raw
0.081	Instant Oatmeal, Quaker, apples & cinnamon prepared w/ boiling water
0.081	Ritz Crackers, Nabisco (Missing Vitamin Data)

0.081	Velveeta cheese, Kraft, pasteurized spread (Missing Data)
0.080	Horseradish, prepared
0.078	Cantaloupe, raw
0.078	Pistachio nuts, dry roasted, no salt
0.073	Parsley, dried (Missing O3FA Data)
0.072	FritoLay Sun Chips, Multi-grain snack, original flavor
0.070	Yogurt, regular low-fat, plain, 12 g protein per 8 oz
0.070	Chili powder
0.070	Mustard seed, yellow
0.070	Cilantro, dried (No O3FA Data)
0.068	Beets, raw
0.067	Culver's shrimp cocktail sauce (Missing Vitamin Data)
0.065	Peanut butter, smooth, USDA Commodity
0.065	Sweet potato, baked in skin, no salt
0.063	Whey protein powder (Low Data)
0.062	Coconut meat, raw
0.062	Salsa, Campbell Pace, Thick & Chunky (Missing Vitamin Data)
0.059	Papayas, raw
0.058	Bagel, plain, unenriched w/ calcium propionate, onion, poppy, sesame (no cream cheese)
0.056	Whole wheat bread, commecially prepared
0.055	Beets, canned, drained solids
0.052	Milk, whole, 3.25% milkfat
0.052	Milk, lowfat, 1%, added Vit A
0.051	Milk, nonfat, added Vit A
0.050	Milk, reduced fat, 2%, added Vit A
0.050	Cashews, dry roasted, no salt
0.049	Strawberries, raw
0.049	Milk, nonfat, Ca fortified
0.048	Turkey, stuffing, mashed potatoes w/ gravy, assorted vegetables, frozen, microwaved
0.048	Chick peas (garbanzo, bengal gram), mature seeds, boiled, no salt
0.048	Carrots, raw, USDA A099
0.047	Peas, frozen, boiled, drained, no salt
0.044	Raspberries, raw
0.043	Avg. Nuts
0.043	White bread, commercially prepared (inlcudes soft crumbs)

0.043	Onion, raw
0.042	Tomato sauce, canned
0.042	Peppers, sweet, red, raw
0.042	Peanuts, dry roasted, no salt, all types
0.042	Macadamia nuts, dry roasted, with salt
0.042	Macadamia nuts, dry roasted, w/out salt
0.041	Greek yogurt
0.041	Pecans, dry roasted, no salt
0.041	Oregano, dried
0.040	Cheerios, General Mills
0.040	Marjoram, dried
0.040	Slice of pizza, fast food, pizza chain, 14", cheese topping, regular crust (No Trans Fat Data)
0.039	Almonds, USDA A256, A264
0.038	Whole wheat bread, prepared from recipe
0.036	Mushrooms, shiitake, cooked, no salt
0.036	Avg. Spice
0.035	Carl's Jr. Italian salad dressing, fat free (Missing Data)
0.035	Potato flour
0.033	Greek style yogurt 150g=2/3 cup (Missing Data)
0.032	Eggplant, boiled, drained, no salt
0.032	Turmeric, ground
0.032	Cream cheese (No Trans Fat Data)
0.032	Corn, sweet, yellow, boiled, drained, no salt
0.030	Light mayo (salad dressing)
0.030	Curry powder
0.030	Poppy seed
0.029	Avg. Vegetables
0.029	Soybeans green, boiled, drained, no salt
0.029	Cheese-flavor puffs or twists, corn-based
0.028	Banquet chicken pot pie, frozen entrée (Missing Data)
0.028	Cabbage, boiled, drained, no salt
0.028	Pretzels, hard, plain, salted
0.028	Cheetos Crunchy cheese-flavored snacks (No O3, 6FA Data)
0.027	Sunflower Seeds, hulled, dry roasted, no salt
0.027	Avg. Herbs

0.027	Cottage cheese, 1% milkfat (No Trans Fat Data)
0.026	Walnuts, USDA A259, A257
0.026	Tomatoes, raw, red, ripe
0.025	Spaghetti squash, winter, boiled w/out salt, drained
0.025	Lemon juice, raw
0.024	Peppers, sweet, green, raw
0.024	Cauliflower, raw
0.023	Brazil nuts, dried, unblanched
0.022	Edamame beans, frozen, prepared
0.020	Iceberg lettuce
0.020	Cinnamon
0.020	Basil, dried
0.020	Cloves, ground
0.020	Cumin seed
0.020	Butternut squash, winter, baked w/out salt, sugar or butter
0.019	Mushrooms, boiled, drained, no salt
0.019	Mushrooms, canned, drained solids
0.019	Radishes, raw
0.019	Asparagus, raw
0.018	Avg. Beans & Lentils
0.018	Lentils, mature seeds, boiled, no salt
0.018	Mushrooms, portabella, raw
0.018	Roll, hard, kaiser
0.017	Egg, whole, cooked, scrambled
0.017	Sage, ground
0.017	Thyme, dried
0.017	Soy sauce (soy & wheat)
0.017	Soy sauce, low sodium (soy & wheat)
0.017	Zucchini, summer squash, w/ skin, boiled w/out salt, drained
0.017	Cucumber, raw w/ peel
0.016	Lima beans, immature, boiled, drained, no salt
0.016	Wheat dinner rolls
0.016	Hotdog, Oscar Mayer Wiener, beef frank (No Trans Fat Data)
0.015	Snap (green string) beans, boiled, drained, no salt
0.015	Flaxseed
0.015	Salami, cooked, beef (No Trans Fat Data)

0.014	Potato, red, baked, flesh & skin
0.014	Mashed potatoes, home-prepared, whole milk & butter added
0.014	Puffed Wheat, Quaker
0.014	Broccoli, boiled, drained, no salt
0.013	White pita bread, enriched
0.013	Ramen noodle soup, chicken flavor, dry
0.013	Banquest Hearty Ones Salisbury Steak Dinner w/ Gravy, Mashed Potatoes and Corn in Seasoned Sauce, frozen meal(Missing Data)
0.013	Pickles, cucumber, dill or kosher dill
0.013	Swiss Cheese (No Trans Fat Data)
0.013	Avg. Leafy Green Vegetables
0.012	Kale, boiled, drained, no salt
0.012	Romaine or cos lettuce
0.012	Potato, baked, flesh & skin, no salt
0.012	Corn chips, extruded, plain
0.011	Mozzarella cheese, part skim (No Trans Fat Data)
0.011	Mayonnaise, soybean oil, w/ salt (salad dressing)
0.011	Swiss chard, boiled, drained, no salt
0.011	Mozzarella cheese, whole milk (No Trans Fat Data)
0.011	Potato, Russet, baked, flesh & skin
0.011	Rye
0.010	Garlic, raw
0.010	Tortilla chips, plain, white corn
0.010	Hot Sauce (ready-to-serve, sauce, pepper or hot)
0.010	Caraway seed
0.010	Celery seed
0.010	Ginger, ground
0.010	Tortilla chips, plain, yellow corn (Missing Vitamin Data)
0.010	Avg. Cheese
0.009	Rice cakes, brown rice, plain
0.009	Popcorn, air-popped
0.009	Parmesan cheese, grated (No Trans Fat Data)
0.009	Sausage, Italian, pork, cooked (No Trans Fat Data)
0.008	Mustard, prepared, yellow
0.008	Pak-choi, boiled, drained, no salt
0.008	Barley (hulled)

0.008	Whole wheat pita bread
0.007	Wild rice, cooked
0.007	Popcorn, microwave, 94% fat free
0.006	Avocado, raw, commercial varieties
0.006	Black pepper
0.006	Spaghetti, cooked, enriched w/out added salt, no sauce
0.005	Cheddar cheese (No Trans Fat Data)
0.005	Provolone cheese (No Trans Fat Data)
0.005	Avg. Cased Meat
0.005	Olives, pickled, canned or bottled, green
0.005	American cheese, pasteurized, w/out disodium phosphate (No Trans Fat Data)
0.005	Blue Cheese (No Trans Fat Data)
0.005	Popcorn, regular butter flavor, microwave, made w/ partially hydrogenated oil (Missing Fats Data)
0.004	Spinach, boiled, drained, no salt
0.004	Whole wheat flour
0.004	New England clam chowder, Campbell's Select (Missing Data)
0.004	Egg noodles, cooked, enriched
0.004	Brown rice, long-grain, cooked
0.004	Potato chips, plain, salted
0.004	Pinto beans, boiled, no salt, mature
0.003	Kidney beans, red, boiled, no salt, mature seeds
0.003	Matzo crackers, plain
0.003	Ricotta cheese, whole milk (No Trans Fat Data)
0.003	Basil, fresh
0.003	Hummus, home prepared
0.003	Chicken noodle soup prepared with equal volume water
0.003	Pretzels, soft
0.003	Oats, unenriched, boiled, w/out salt
0.002	White flour, white, all-purpose, enriched, bleached
0.002	Sesame sticks, wheat-based, salted
0.002	McDonald's French Fries
0.001	Swanson chicken broth, 99% Fat Free
0.001	Parboiled rice, white, long-grain, enriched, cooked
0.001	Millet, cooked
0.001	Pastrami luncheon meat, beef, cured (No Trans Fat Data)

0.001	Cream of Wheat, instant, prepared with water and salt
0.001	Grits, corn, white, regular, quick, enriched, cooked with water, with salt
0.001	White rice, long-grain, regular, cooked
0.001	White rice, glutinous, cooked

Starch

Note: In this case, "starch" was calculated by "total carbs – fiber – sugar," therefore, the values below may capture "carbs" that were not accounted for by "fiber" and "sugar."

Starch, g/SS	Food
0.905	Corn starch (Missing O3FA Data)
0.804	Matzo crackers, plain
0.764	Rice cakes, brown rice, plain
0.750	Rice Krispies, Kellogg's
0.741	Corn Flakes, Kellogg's
0.738	Potato flour
0.735	Pretzels, hard, whole-wheat (Missing Sugar Data)
0.734	Pretzels, hard, plain, salted
0.734	White flour, white, all-purpose, enriched, bleached
0.674	Pretzels, soft
0.656	Puffed Wheat, Quaker
0.625	Popcorn, air-popped
0.617	Popcorn, microwave, 94% fat free
0.616	Tortilla chips, plain, yellow corn (Missing Vitamin Data)
0.615	Saffron (Missing Data)
0.606	Cheerios, General Mills
0.600	Whole wheat flour
0.599	Ramen noodle soup, chicken flavor, dry
0.593	Tortilla chips, plain, white corn
0.575	Wheaties, General Mills
0.567	Corn chips, extruded, plain
0.558	Kraft macaroni & cheese dinner, original, unprepared (Missing Data)
0.554	Oats
0.553	Barley (hulled)
0.541	Rye
0.537	Pumpkin/Squash Seeds, dry roasted, no salt (Missing Vitamin & Se Data)
0.533	FritoLay Sun Chips, Multi-grain snack, original flavor
0.531	Ritz Crackers, Nabisco (Missing Vitamin Data)
0.522	White pita bread, enriched
0.520	Post Honey Bunches of Oats w/ Almonds (Missing Data)

0.509	Cheetos Crunchy cheese-flavored snacks (No O3, 6FA Data)
0.503	Frosted Flakes, Kellogg's
0.501	Cocoa Krispies, Kellogg's (No O3FA Data)
0.500	Allspice (Missing Data)
0.498	High-fructose corn syrup
0.490	Bay leaf (Missing Data)
0.486	Roll, hard, kaiser
0.481	Honeycomb cereal, Post, Kraft (low data)
0.476	Cheese-flavor puffs or twists, corn-based
0.468	Whole wheat pita bread
0.468	Apple Jacks, Kellogg's
0.453	Bagel, plain, unenriched w/ calcium propionate, onion, poppy, sesame (no cream cheese)
0.453	Popcorn, regular butter flavor, microwave, made w/ partially hydrogenated oil (Missing Fats Data)
0.450	Potato chips, plain, salted
0.439	White bread, commercially prepared (inlcudes soft crumbs)
0.439	Bran Flakes, single brand
0.435	Sesame sticks, wheat-based, salted
0.429	Peanut Butter Cap'n Crunch, Quaker
0.428	Tarragon, dried (Missing Data)
0.427	Cinnamon Toast Crunch cereal, ready-to-eat, General Mills
0.420	Dill weed, dried (Missing Data)
0.416	Whole wheat bread, prepared from recipe
0.413	Corn Pops, Kellogg's
0.406	Wheat dinner rolls
0.406	Turmeric, ground
0.400	Cardamom (Missing Data)
0.394	Froot Loops, General Mills
0.385	Cap'n Crunch, Quaker
0.383	Lucky Charms, General Mills
0.380	Cap'n Crunch with Crunch Berries, Quaker
0.377	Black pepper
0.375	Granola bar, soft, uncoated, chocolate chip
0.370	Golden Crisp, Post, Kraft
0.364	Kellogg's Raisin Bran
0.352	Kellogg's Nutri-Grain Cereal Bars, fruit-filled

0.350	Cocoa Puffs, General Mills
0.350	Anise seed (Missing Sugar, Vitamin, O3FA data)
0.350	Cilantro, dried (No O3FA Data)
0.347	McDonald's French Fries
0.330	Fenugreek seed (Missing Vitamin & O3, 6FA Data)
0.310	Cumin seed
0.300	Mace, ground (Missing Data)
0.299	Garlic, raw
0.293	Honey Smacks, Kellogg's
0.289	Whole wheat bread, commecially prepared
0.285	Spaghetti, cooked, enriched w/out added salt, no sauce
0.280	Celery seed
0.277	White rice, long-grain, regular, cooked
0.269	Slice of pizza, fast food, pizza chain, 14", cheese topping, regular crust (No Trans Fat Data)
0.263	White rice, long-grain, pre-cooked or instant, prepared (Missing O3FA Data)
0.260	Cinnamon
0.252	Thyme, dried
0.251	Parboiled rice, white, long-grain, enriched, cooked
0.250	Cloves, ground
0.247	Cashews, dry roasted, no salt
0.247	Soybeans (aka soy nuts) mature, dry roasted (Missing Sugar and Vitamin Data)
0.239	Rice noodles, cooked (Missing Sugar & Unsaturated Fat Data)
0.236	Egg noodles, cooked, enriched
0.233	Avg. Spice
0.222	Millet, cooked
0.220	Curry powder
0.219	Whey protein powder (Low Data)
0.215	Rosemary, dried (Missing Data)
0.208	Brown rice, long-grain, cooked
0.207	Apricot jam and preserves
0.207	Popcorn, caramel-coated without peanuts
0.201	White rice, glutinous, cooked
0.195	Avg. Herbs
0.193	Cake, snack cakes, crème-filled, chocolate with frosting

0.191	Corn, sweet, yellow, boiled, drained, no salt
0.190	Basil, dried
0.188	Wild rice, cooked
0.187	Sage, ground
0.185	Quinoa, cooked
0.182	Chick peas (garbanzo, bengal gram), mature seeds, canned
0.181	Potato, Russet, baked, flesh & skin
0.178	Potato, baked, flesh & skin, no salt
0.175	Oregano, dried
0.170	Marjoram, dried
0.168	Pinto beans, boiled, no salt, mature
0.167	Lima beans, immature, boiled, drained, no salt
0.166	Culver's shrimp cocktail sauce (Missing Vitamin Data)
0.165	Raisins, seedless
0.164	Potato, red, baked, flesh & skin
0.159	Hummus, home prepared
0.154	Banana chips
0.151	Kidney beans, red, boiled, no salt, mature seeds
0.150	Chick peas (garbanzo, bengal gram), mature seeds, boiled, no salt
0.150	Ginger, ground
0.140	Parsley, dried (Missing O3FA Data)
0.140	Chili powder
0.139	Mashed potatoes, home-prepared, whole milk & butter added
0.135	Banquet chicken pot pie, frozen entrée (Missing Data)
0.130	Mustard seed, yellow
0.130	Coriander seed (Missing Data)
0.125	Grits, corn, white, regular, quick, enriched, cooked with water, with salt
0.124	Cream of Wheat, instant, prepared with water and salt
0.120	Fennel seed (Missing Vitamin & O3FA Data)
0.118	Peanut butter, smooth, USDA Commodity
0.116	Oats, unenriched, boiled, w/out salt
0.110	Caraway seed
0.109	Sweet potato, baked in skin, no salt
0.105	Lentils, mature seeds, boiled, no salt
0.104	Thyme, fresh (Missing Data)

0.103	Avg. Beans & Lentils
0.102	Sunflower Seeds, hulled, dry roasted, no salt
0.102	Turkey, stuffing, mashed potatoes w/ gravy, assorted vegetables, frozen, microwaved
0.100	Mustard, Subway, yellow & deli brown (Missing Vitamin Data)
0.096	Black beans, mature seeds, canned
0.095	Pistachio nuts, dry roasted, no salt
0.093	Peanuts, dry roasted, no salt, all types
0.088	Mushrooms, shiitake, cooked, no salt
0.081	Banana, raw
0.080	Paprika
0.079	Dark chocolate candies, 60-69% cacao solids (Missing Vitamin Data)
0.079	Instant Oatmeal, Quaker, apples & cinnamon prepared w/ boiling water
0.078	Oysters, eastern, wild, cooked, moist heat
0.078	Candy bar, Snickers (King Size)
0.075	Syrups, maple
0.073	Avg. Nuts
0.071	Butternut squash, winter, baked w/out salt, sugar or butter
0.070	Acerola (West Indian cherry), raw (Missing Sugar and Vitamin Data)
0.066	Rosemarry, fresh (Missing Data)
0.065	Banquest Hearty Ones Salisbury Steak Dinner w/ Gravy, Mashed Potatoes and Corn in Seasoned Sauce, frozen meal(Missing Data)
0.061	Chia seeds, dried (Missing Sugar and Vitamin Data)
0.060	Soy sauce, low sodium (soy & wheat)
0.057	Lemon juice, raw
0.056	Poppy seed
0.056	Bologna, chicken, pork, beef
0.056	Salsa, USDA Commodity (Missing Sugar and Vitamin Data)
0.056	Almonds, USDA A256, A264
0.054	Beef sticks, smoked (No Trans Fat Data)
0.052	Light mayo (salad dressing)
0.051	Soy sauce (soy & wheat)
0.051	Clams, mixed species, cooked in moist heat
0.049	New England clam chowder, Campbell's Select (Missing Data)
0.045	Milk chocolate candies (No Trans Fat Data)
0.044	Walnuts, USDA A259, A257

0.041	Peas, frozen, boiled, drained, no salt
0.041	Swiss Cheese (No Trans Fat Data)
0.039	Oysters, eastern, wild, raw
0.035	Carl's Jr. Italian salad dressing, fat free (Missing Data)
0.034	Onion, raw
0.034	Weight Watchers Smart Ones Chicken Enchiladas Suiza, Sour Cream w/ Cheese frozen entrée (Missing Data)
0.033	Sausage, Italian, pork, cooked (No Trans Fat Data)
0.032	Parmesan cheese, grated (No Trans Fat Data)
0.031	Snap (green string) beans, boiled, drained, no salt
0.030	Spam, Hormel (Missing Data)
0.028	Chocolate-flavored hazelnut spread (No Trans Fat Data)
0.028	Edamame beans, frozen, prepared
0.027	Ricotta cheese, whole milk (No Trans Fat Data)
0.025	Spaghetti squash, winter, boiled w/out salt, drained
0.025	Broccoli, boiled, drained, no salt
0.025	Chicken noodle soup prepared with equal volume water
0.024	Brazil nuts, dried, unblanched
0.024	Eggplant, boiled, drained, no salt
0.024	Kale, boiled, drained, no salt
0.021	Ketchup
0.021	Blueberries, raw
0.021	Mayonnaise, soybean oil, w/ salt (salad dressing)
0.021	Papayas, raw
0.020	Carrots, raw, USDA A099
0.020	Margarine (vegetable oil spread, 70% fat, soybean & partially hydrogenated soybean, stick)
0.019	Avg. Cheese
0.018	Pineapple, raw, all varieties
0.018	Blue Cheese (No Trans Fat Data)
0.018	Mushrooms, portabella, raw
0.017	Ice creams, vanilla (No Trans Fat Data)
0.017	Velveeta cheese, Kraft, pasteurized spread (Missing Data)
0.017	Mozzarella cheese, part skim (No Trans Fat Data)
0.017	Cranberry juice cocktail, bottled
0.017	Grapes, red or green, European type such as Thompson seedless, raw
0.016	Spearmint, fresh (Missing Data)

0.016	Salami, dry or hard, pork (No Trans Fat Data)
0.016	Provolone cheese (No Trans Fat Data)
0.015	Avg. Fruit
0.015	Avg. Cased Meat
0.015	Bacon (pork), cured, cooked, pan-fried
0.015	Apple Juice, canned or bottled, unsweetened
0.015	Cucumber, raw w/ peel
0.014	Brown sugars
0.014	Teriyaki sauce, ready-to-serve
0.013	Lobster, northern, cooked in moist heat
0.013	McDonald's barbeque sauce
0.012	Mushrooms, boiled, drained, no salt
0.012	Macadamia nuts, dry roasted, w/out salt
0.012	Mustard, prepared, yellow
0.012	Hotdog, Oscar Mayer Wiener, beef frank (No Trans Fat Data)
0.012	Soybeans green, boiled, drained, no salt
0.012	Mozzarella cheese, whole milk (No Trans Fat Data)
0.012	Sprite
0.011	Avocado, raw, commercial varieties
0.011	American cheese, pasteurized, w/out disodium phosphate (No Trans Fat Data)
0.011	Avg. Leafy Green Vegetables
0.011	Raspberries, raw
0.010	Cherries, sweet, raw
0.010	Pomegranate, raw
0.010	Hot Sauce (ready-to-serve, sauce, pepper or hot)
0.010	Apple, raw, with skin A343
0.010	Macadamia nuts, dry roasted, with salt
0.009	Swiss chard, boiled, drained, no salt
0.009	Spinach, boiled, drained, no salt
0.009	Zucchini, summer squash, w/ skin, boiled w/out salt, drained
0.009	Cream cheese (No Trans Fat Data)
0.009	Strawberries, raw
0.008	Cabbage, boiled, drained, no salt
0.008	Basil, fresh
0.008	Avg. Vegetables

0.008	Mushrooms, canned, drained solids
0.008	Cheddar cheese (No Trans Fat Data)
0.005	Peppers, sweet, green, raw
0.005	Egg, whole, cooked, scrambled
0.005	Avg. Seafood
0.004	Mangos, raw
0.004	Bologna, lebanon, beef (No O3FA Data)
0.004	Cauliflower, raw
0.004	Salami, cooked, beef (No Trans Fat Data)
0.004	Grape Juice, canned or bottled, unsweetened
0.003	Ice cream, soft-serve, french vanilla (No Trans Fat Data)
0.003	McDonald's spicy buffalo sauce
0.002	Chamomile Tea (No O3FA & O6FA Data)
0.002	Pecans, dry roasted, no salt
0.002	Pickles, cucumber, dill or kosher dill
0.001	Flaxseed
0.001	Sugars, granulated (sucrose)
0.001	Cantaloupe, raw
0.001	Tomatoes, raw, red, ripe
0.001	Ginger Ale

Protein

Protein, g/SS	Food
62.500	Whey protein powder (Low Data)
61.300	Pork-skins, plain
39.593	Soybeans (aka soy nuts) mature, dry roasted (Missing Sugar and Vitamin Data)
38.500	Parmesan cheese, grated (No Trans Fat Data)
38.300	Bacon (pork), cured, cooked, pan-fried
31.000	Chicken, broilers or fryers, breast, meat only (no skin), roasted
30.100	Turkey, fryer-roaster, breast meat only, roasted
29.300	Beef, eye of round, separable lean only, trimmed to 0" fat, all grades, roasted [cube steak]
29.150	Avg. Lean Meat
28.900	Anchovies, European, canned in oil, drained solids
27.400	Ground turkey, cooked
27.100	Corned beef luncheon meat, beef, cured, canned (No Trans Fat Data)
26.894	Swiss Cheese (No Trans Fat Data)
26.294	Red snapper, cooked, dry heat
26.200	Pork tenderloin lean, roasted, URMIS 3358
26.100	Tilapia, cooked in dry heat
25.700	Hamburger patty, 80/20 ground chuck beef, broiled
25.606	Provolone cheese (No Trans Fat Data)
25.515	Tuna fish, light, canned in water without salt, drained solids
25.500	Clams, mixed species, cooked in moist heat
25.455	Salmon, Atlantic, wild, cooked in dry heat
25.377	Swordfish, cooked in dry heat
25.000	Mustard seed, yellow
25.000	Monterey Jack cheese (Missing Data)
24.924	Cheddar cheese (No Trans Fat Data)
24.321	T-bone steak, short loin, beef trimmed to 1/8" fat, all grades, broiled
24.300	Mozzarella cheese, part skim (No Trans Fat Data)
24.173	Flounder (sole), cooked in dry heat
24.077	Avg. Seafood
23.699	Peanuts, dry roasted, no salt, all types
23.605	Tuna fish, white, canned in water without salt, drained solids

23.500	Whiting, mixed species, cooked in dry heat
23.200	Scallops (bay & sea), steamed
23.000	Fenugreek seed (Missing Vitamin & O3, 6FA Data)
22.800	Tarragon, dried (Missing Data)
22.700	Pepperoni, pork, beef
22.566	Salami, dry or hard, pork (No Trans Fat Data)
22.400	Parsley, dried (Missing O3FA Data)
22.200	American cheese, pasteurized, w/out disodium phosphate (No Trans Fat Data)
22.143	Mozzarella cheese, whole milk (No Trans Fat Data)
22.102	Avg. Cheese
22.000	Cilantro, dried (No O3FA Data)
21.938	Peanut butter, smooth, USDA Commodity
21.800	Pastrami luncheon meat, beef, cured (No Trans Fat Data)
21.500	Beef sticks, smoked (No Trans Fat Data)
21.400	Blue Cheese (No Trans Fat Data)
21.382	Pistachio nuts, dry roasted, no salt
21.189	Almonds, USDA A256, A264
20.900	Shrimp, mixed species, cooked in moist heat
20.483	Lobster, northern, cooked in moist heat
20.000	Caraway seed
20.000	Dill weed, dried (Missing Data)
19.297	Sunflower Seeds, hulled, dry roased, no salt
19.100	Sausage, Italian, pork, cooked (No Trans Fat Data)
19.000	Bologna, lebanon, beef (No O3FA Data)
18.558	Avg. Cased Meat
18.500	Pumpkin/Squash Seeds, dry roasted, no salt (Missing Vitamin & Se Data)
18.300	Flaxseed
18.000	Celery seed
18.000	Cumin seed
18.000	Poppy seed
18.000	Anise seed (Missing Sugar, Vitamin, O3FA data)
17.500	Crayfish, mixed species, farmed, cooked in moist heat
16.923	Oats
16.860	Soybeans green, boiled, drained, no salt
16.300	Puffed Wheat, Quaker

16.300	Velveeta cheese, Kraft, pasteurized spread (Missing Data)
16.200	Kraft macaroni & cheese dinner, original, unprepared (Missing Data)
16.000	Fennel seed (Missing Vitamin & O3FA Data)
15.691	Avg. Nuts
15.600	Chia seeds, dried (Missing Sugar and Vitamin Data)
15.328	Cashews, dry roasted, no salt
15.214	Walnuts, USDA A259, A257
14.800	Paprika
14.734	Rye
14.286	Brazil nuts, dried, unblanched
14.100	Oysters, eastern, wild, cooked, moist heat
14.000	Basil, dried
13.667	Whole wheat flour
13.600	Avg. Spice
13.200	Spam, Hormel (Missing Data)
13.000	Whole wheat bread, commecially prepared
13.000	Curry powder
13.000	Marjoram, dried
12.900	Popcorn, air-popped
12.600	Salami, cooked, beef (No Trans Fat Data)
12.500	Barley (hulled)
12.389	Cottage cheese, 1% milkfat (No Trans Fat Data)
12.000	Chili powder
12.000	Coriander seed (Missing Data)
11.942	Slice of pizza, fast food, pizza chain, 14", cheese topping, regular crust (No Trans Fat Data)
11.540	Avg. Herbs
11.400	Saffron (Missing Data)
11.300	Cheerios, General Mills
11.300	Ricotta cheese, whole milk (No Trans Fat Data)
11.300	Bologna, chicken, pork, beef
11.300	Hotdog, Oscar Mayer Wiener, beef frank (No Trans Fat Data)
11.100	Egg, whole, cooked, scrambled
11.100	Pretzels, hard, whole-wheat (Missing Sugar Data)
11.000	Oregano, dried
11.000	Black pepper

11.000	Cardamom (Missing Data)
10.903	Edamame beans, frozen, prepared
10.900	Sesame sticks, wheat-based, salted
10.700	Popcorn, microwave, 94% fat free
10.700	Ramen noodle soup, chicken flavor, dry
10.600	Sage, ground
10.588	Greek yogurt
10.534	Bagel, plain, unenriched w/ calcium propionate, onion, poppy, sesame (no cream cheese)
10.320	White flour, white, all-purpose, enriched, bleached
10.300	Pretzels, hard, plain, salted
10.000	Matzo crackers, plain
10.000	Wheaties, General Mills
9.900	Roll, hard, kaiser
9.800	Whole wheat pita bread
9.500	Pecans, dry roasted, no salt
9.400	Bran Flakes, single brand
9.100	White pita bread, enriched
9.100	Thyme, dried
9.040	Lentils, mature seeds, boiled, no salt
9.006	Pinto beans, boiled, no salt, mature
8.841	Chick peas (garbanzo, bengal gram), mature seeds, boiled, no salt
8.700	Popcorn, regular butter flavor, microwave, made w/ partially hydrogenated oil (Missing Fats Data)
8.644	Kidney beans, red, boiled, no salt, mature seeds
8.600	Wheat dinner rolls
8.600	Kellogg's Raisin Bran
8.400	Whole wheat bread, prepared from recipe
8.200	Rice cakes, brown rice, plain
8.182	Pretzels, soft
8.001	Avg. Beans & Lentils
8.000	Post Honey Bunches of Oats w/ Almonds (Missing Data)
8.000	Bay leaf (Missing Data)
7.900	FritoLay Sun Chips, Multi-grain snack, original flavor
7.886	Hummus, home prepared
7.803	Macadamia nuts, dry roasted, with salt
7.803	Macadamia nuts, dry roasted, w/out salt

7.800	Tortilla chips, plain, white corn
7.800	Turmeric, ground
7.679	Milk chocolate candies (No Trans Fat Data)
7.600	White bread, commercially prepared (inlcudes soft crumbs)
7.522	Candy bar, Snickers (King Size)
7.333	Greek style yogurt 150g=2/3 cup (Missing Data)
7.200	Ritz Crackers, Nabisco (Missing Vitamin Data)
7.200	Tortilla chips, plain, yellow corn (Missing Vitamin Data)
7.100	Peanut Butter Cap'n Crunch, Quaker
7.056	Oysters, eastern, wild, raw
7.000	Lucky Charms, General Mills
7.000	Mace, ground (Missing Data)
6.961	Turkey, stuffing, mashed potatoes w/ gravy, assorted vegetables, frozen, microwaved
6.875	Potato flour
6.824	Lima beans, immature, boiled, drained, no salt
6.800	Rice Krispies, Kellogg's
6.600	Corn Flakes, Kellogg's
6.564	Potato chips, plain, salted
6.400	Honey Smacks, Kellogg's
6.324	Garlic, raw
6.275	Soy sauce (soy & wheat)
6.161	Dark chocolate candies, 60-69% cacao solids (Missing Vitamin Data)
6.010	Corn chips, extruded, plain
6.000	Cloves, ground
6.000	Allspice (Missing Data)
6.000	Nutmeg, ground (Missing O3FA Data)
5.948	Cream cheese (No Trans Fat Data)
5.938	Teriyaki sauce, ready-to-serve
5.833	Black beans, mature seeds, canned
5.800	Cheese-flavor puffs or twists, corn-based
5.786	Spaghetti, cooked, enriched w/out added salt, no sauce
5.606	Banquet chicken pot pie, frozen entrée (Missing Data)
5.600	Granola bar, soft, uncoated, chocolate chip
5.600	Thyme, fresh (Missing Data)
5.500	Golden Crisp, Post, Kraft

5.400	Chocolate-flavored hazelnut spread (No Trans Fat Data)
5.300	Cinnamon Toast Crunch cereal, ready-to-eat, General Mills
5.294	Weight Watchers Smart Ones Chicken Enchiladas Suiza, Sour Cream w/ Cheese frozen entrée (Missing Data)
5.265	Yogurt, regular low-fat, plain, 12 g protein per 8 oz
5.200	Cocoa Krispies, Kellogg's (No O3FA Data)
5.200	Honeycomb cereal, Post, Kraft (low data)
5.176	Soy sauce, low sodium (soy & wheat)
5.138	Peas, frozen, boiled, drained, no salt
5.132	Banquet Hearty Ones Salisbury Steak Dinner w/ Gravy, Mashed Potatoes and Corn in Seasoned Sauce, frozen meal(Missing Data)
5.000	Chick peas (garbanzo, bengal gram), mature seeds, canned
4.900	Rosemary, dried (Missing Data)
4.563	Egg noodles, cooked, enriched
4.400	Kellogg's Nutri-Grain Cereal Bars, fruit-filled
4.400	Cap'n Crunch, Quaker
4.400	Cap'n Crunch with Crunch Berries, Quaker
4.378	Quinoa, cooked
4.378	Mustard, prepared, yellow
4.300	Frosted Flakes, Kellogg's
4.200	Apple Jacks, Kellogg's
4.100	Ice cream, soft-serve, french vanilla (No Trans Fat Data)
4.000	Cinnamon
3.963	Wild rice, cooked
3.846	McDonald's French Fries
3.800	Popcorn, caramel-coated without peanuts
3.700	Corn Pops, Kellogg's
3.600	Cake, snack cakes, crème-filled, chocolate with frosting
3.506	Millet, cooked
3.500	Ice creams, vanilla (No Trans Fat Data)
3.401	Milk, nonfat, Ca fortified
3.400	Froot Loops, General Mills
3.388	Milk, nonfat, added Vit A
3.361	Milk, lowfat, 1%, added Vit A
3.325	Coconut meat, raw
3.320	Milk, reduced fat, 2%, added Vit A
3.300	Cocoa Puffs, General Mills

3.300	Rosemarry, fresh (Missing Data)
3.300	Spearmint, fresh (Missing Data)
3.293	Corn, sweet, yellow, boiled, drained, no salt
3.238	Milk, whole, 3.25% milkfat
3.200	Basil, fresh
3.091	Raisins, seedless
3.000	Ginger, ground
2.944	Spinach, boiled, drained, no salt
2.911	Parboiled rice, white, long-grain, enriched, cooked
2.800	Cheetos Crunchy cheese-flavored snacks (No O3, 6FA Data)
2.658	White rice, long-grain, regular, cooked
2.642	Potato, Russet, baked, flesh & skin
2.564	Brown rice, long-grain, cooked
2.521	Oats, unenriched, boiled, w/out salt
2.508	Potato, baked, flesh & skin, no salt
2.500	Mushrooms, portabella, raw
2.449	New England clam chowder, Campbell's Select (Missing Data)
2.393	Broccoli, boiled, drained, no salt
2.308	Potato, red, baked, flesh & skin
2.300	Banana chips
2.182	White rice, long-grain, pre-cooked or instant, prepared (Missing O3FA Data)
2.179	Mushrooms, boiled, drained, no salt
2.164	Asparagus, raw
2.011	White rice, glutinous, cooked
2.000	Cauliflower, raw
2.000	Sweet potato, baked in skin, no salt
1.990	Avocado, raw, commercial varieties
1.923	Kale, boiled, drained, no salt
1.920	Snap (green string) beans, boiled, drained, no salt
1.900	Margarine, industrial, non-dairy, cottonseed, soy oil (partially hydrogenated), for flaky pastries
1.891	Avg. Leafy Green Vegetables
1.886	Swiss chard, boiled, drained, no salt
1.859	Mushrooms, canned, drained solids
1.857	Mashed potatoes, home-prepared, whole milk & butter added
1.826	Cream of Wheat, instant, prepared with water and salt

1.812	Instant Oatmeal, Quaker, apples & cinnamon prepared w/ boiling water
1.750	Ketchup
1.700	Pomegranate, raw
1.618	Beets, raw
1.588	Pak-choi, boiled, drained, no salt
1.586	Mushrooms, shiitake, cooked, no salt
1.500	McDonald's barbeque sauce
1.500	Salsa, USDA Commodity (Missing Sugar and Vitamin Data)
1.405	Grits, corn, white, regular, quick, enriched, cooked with water, with salt
1.306	Tomato sauce, canned
1.300	Cabbage, boiled, drained, no salt
1.250	Chicken noodle soup prepared with equal volume water
1.220	Raspberries, raw
1.207	Avg. Vegetables
1.200	Romaine or cos lettuce
1.200	Horseradish, prepared
1.125	Onion, raw
1.103	Banana, raw
1.087	Cherries, sweet, raw
1.007	Peppers, sweet, red, raw
1.000	Olives, pickled, canned or bottled, green
1.000	Hot Sauce (ready-to-serve, sauce, pepper or hot)
0.944	Orange, raw, all commercial varieties
0.938	Carrots, raw, USDA A099
0.918	Beets, canned, drained solids
0.914	Peaches, raw
0.909	Mayonnaise, soybean oil, w/ salt (salad dressing)
0.909	Rice noodles, cooked (Missing Sugar & Unsaturated Fat Data)
0.900	Iceberg lettuce
0.900	Light mayo (salad dressing)
0.882	Cantaloupe, raw
0.878	Butternut squash, winter, baked w/out salt, sugar or butter
0.872	Tomatoes, raw, red, ripe
0.872	Peppers, sweet, green, raw
0.849	Avg. Fruit

0.837	Butter, salted (No Trans Fat Data)
0.800	Eggplant, boiled, drained, no salt
0.728	Grapes, red or green, European type such as Thompson seedless, raw
0.700	Blueberries, raw
0.700	Apricot jam and preserves
0.690	Radishes, raw
0.667	Zucchini, summer squash, w/ skin, boiled w/out salt, drained
0.658	Strawberries, raw
0.645	Spaghetti squash, winter, boiled w/out salt, drained
0.643	Papayas, raw
0.581	Pickles, cucumber, dill or kosher dill
0.545	Pineapple, raw, all varieties
0.529	Swanson chicken broth, 99% Fat Free
0.500	McDonald's spicy buffalo sauce
0.497	Pineapple, canned, juice pack, drained
0.485	Mangos, raw
0.410	Lemon juice, raw
0.356	Grape Juice, canned or bottled, unsweetened
0.295	Honey
0.269	Apple, raw, with skin A343
0.234	Corn starch (Missing O3FA Data)
0.136	Brown sugars
0.115	Apple Juice, canned or bottled, unsweetened
0.110	Coffee, brewed from grounds w/ tap water, no sugar or cream (No O3FA Data)
0.058	Sprite

Protein/Calories

Please note that "calories" represents total calories, and are not distinguished by the different *type of calories*. Also, serving size is constant in regards to the values taken for protein and calories for each food.

Protein, g/Calories	Food
0.223	Turkey, fryer-roaster, breast meat only, roasted
0.220	Tuna fish, light, canned in water without salt, drained solids
0.211	Shrimp, mixed species, cooked in moist heat
0.209	Lobster, northern, cooked in moist heat
0.207	Scallops (bay & sea), steamed
0.206	Flounder (sole), cooked in dry heat
0.205	Red snapper, cooked, dry heat
0.204	Tilapia, cooked in dry heat
0.203	Whiting, mixed species, cooked in dry heat
0.201	Crayfish, mixed species, farmed, cooked in moist heat
0.194	Avg. Lean Meat
0.189	Avg. Seafood
0.188	Chicken, broilers or fryers, breast, meat only (no skin), roasted
0.185	Tuna fish, white, canned in water without salt, drained solids
0.183	Pork tenderloin lean, roasted, URMIS 3358
0.181	Beef, eye of round, separable lean only, trimmed to 0" fat, all grades, roasted [cube steak]
0.180	Greek yogurt
0.172	Clams, mixed species, cooked in moist heat
0.172	Cottage cheese, 1% milkfat (No Trans Fat Data)
0.164	Swordfish, cooked in dry heat
0.154	Whey protein powder (Low Data)
0.150	Coffee, brewed from grounds w/ tap water, no sugar or cream (No O3FA Data)
0.149	Pastrami luncheon meat, beef, cured (No Trans Fat Data)
0.140	Salmon, Atlantic, wild, cooked in dry heat
0.139	Basil, fresh
0.138	Anchovies, European, canned in oil, drained solids
0.135	Pak-choi, boiled, drained, no salt
0.133	Swanson chicken broth, 99% Fat Free

0.129	Spinach, boiled, drained, no salt
0.119	Soy sauce (soy & wheat)
0.117	Ground turkey, cooked
0.113	Pork-skins, plain
0.110	Bologna, lebanon, beef (No O3FA Data)
0.108	Corned beef luncheon meat, beef, cured, canned (No Trans Fat Data)
0.107	Asparagus, raw
0.104	Oysters, eastern, wild, raw
0.103	Oysters, eastern, wild, cooked, moist heat
0.100	Milk, nonfat, added Vit A
0.098	Soy sauce, low sodium (soy & wheat)
0.098	Milk, nonfat, Ca fortified
0.097	Soybeans green, boiled, drained, no salt
0.096	Mushrooms, portabella, raw
0.096	Mozzarella cheese, part skim (No Trans Fat Data)
0.095	Hamburger patty, 80/20 ground chuck beef, broiled
0.094	Swiss chard, boiled, drained, no salt
0.091	Hot Sauce (ready-to-serve, sauce, pepper or hot)
0.089	Edamame beans, frozen, prepared
0.089	Parmesan cheese, grated (No Trans Fat Data)
0.089	Avg. Leafy Green Vegetables
0.088	Soybeans (aka soy nuts) mature, dry roasted (Missing Sugar and Vitamin Data)
0.087	T-bone steak, short loin, beef trimmed to 1/8" fat, all grades, broiled
0.085	Greek style yogurt 150g=2/3 cup (Missing Data)
0.084	Yogurt, regular low-fat, plain, 12 g protein per 8 oz
0.081	Parsley, dried (Missing O3FA Data)
0.080	Milk, lowfat, 1%, added Vit A
0.080	Cauliflower, raw
0.079	Dill weed, dried (Missing Data)
0.079	Cilantro, dried (No O3FA Data)
0.078	Lentils, mature seeds, boiled, no salt
0.077	Tarragon, dried (Missing Data)
0.077	Mushrooms, boiled, drained, no salt
0.075	Spearmint, fresh (Missing Data)

0.074	Mushrooms, canned, drained solids
0.074	Mozzarella cheese, whole milk (No Trans Fat Data)
0.073	Provolone cheese (No Trans Fat Data)
0.072	Bacon (pork), cured, cooked, pan-fried
0.071	Fenugreek seed (Missing Vitamin & O3, 6FA Data)
0.071	Swiss Cheese (No Trans Fat Data)
0.071	Romaine or cos lettuce
0.070	Monterey Jack cheese (Missing Data)
0.069	Kale, boiled, drained, no salt
0.068	Broccoli, boiled, drained, no salt
0.068	Kidney beans, red, boiled, no salt, mature seeds
0.067	Avg. Cased Meat
0.067	Teriyaki sauce, ready-to-serve
0.067	Avg. Beans & Lentils
0.066	Egg, whole, cooked, scrambled
0.066	Milk, reduced fat, 2%, added Vit A
0.066	Peas, frozen, boiled, drained, no salt
0.065	Mustard, prepared, yellow
0.065	Ricotta cheese, whole milk (No Trans Fat Data)
0.064	Iceberg lettuce
0.064	Black beans, mature seeds, canned
0.063	Avg. Cheese
0.063	Pinto beans, boiled, no salt, mature
0.062	Cheddar cheese (No Trans Fat Data)
0.061	Blue Cheese (No Trans Fat Data)
0.060	Caraway seed
0.059	American cheese, pasteurized, w/out disodium phosphate (No Trans Fat Data)
0.057	Cabbage, boiled, drained, no salt
0.056	Basil, dried
0.056	Sausage, Italian, pork, cooked (No Trans Fat Data)
0.056	Lima beans, immature, boiled, drained, no salt
0.055	Thyme, fresh (Missing Data)
0.055	Salami, dry or hard, pork (No Trans Fat Data)
0.055	Snap (green string) beans, boiled, drained, no salt
0.054	Turkey, stuffing, mashed potatoes w/ gravy, assorted vegetables, frozen, microwaved

0.054	Tomato sauce, canned
0.054	Milk, whole, 3.25% milkfat
0.054	Chick peas (garbanzo, bengal gram), mature seeds, boiled, no salt
0.054	Velveeta cheese, Kraft, pasteurized spread (Missing Data)
0.053	Anise seed (Missing Sugar, Vitamin, O3FA data)
0.053	Mustard seed, yellow
0.053	Whole wheat bread, commecially prepared
0.051	Paprika
0.050	Chicken noodle soup prepared with equal volume water
0.048	Salami, cooked, beef (No Trans Fat Data)
0.048	Tomatoes, raw, red, ripe
0.048	Cumin seed
0.048	Marjoram, dried
0.047	Pickles, cucumber, dill or kosher dill
0.046	Fennel seed (Missing Vitamin & O3FA Data)
0.046	Pepperoni, pork, beef
0.046	Celery seed
0.045	Slice of pizza, fast food, pizza chain, 14", cheese topping, regular crust (No Trans Fat Data)
0.045	Hummus, home prepared
0.045	Puffed Wheat, Quaker
0.044	Avg. Vegetables
0.044	Rye
0.044	Kraft macaroni & cheese dinner, original, unprepared (Missing Data)
0.043	Oats
0.043	Weight Watchers Smart Ones Chicken Enchiladas Suiza, Sour Cream w/ Cheese frozen entrée (Missing Data)
0.043	Peppers, sweet, green, raw
0.043	Black pepper
0.043	Spam, Hormel (Missing Data)
0.042	Garlic, raw
0.042	Radishes, raw
0.042	Chick peas (garbanzo, bengal gram), mature seeds, canned
0.042	Salsa, USDA Commodity (Missing Sugar and Vitamin Data)

0.042	Bologna, chicken, pork, beef
0.041	Pumpkin/Squash Seeds, dry roasted, no salt (Missing Vitamin & Se Data)
0.041	Zucchini, summer squash, w/ skin, boiled w/out salt, drained
0.041	Avg. Herbs
0.041	Peanuts, dry roasted, no salt, all types
0.040	Whole wheat flour
0.040	Coriander seed (Missing Data)
0.040	Curry powder
0.040	Avg. Spice
0.039	Wild rice, cooked
0.039	Beef sticks, smoked (No Trans Fat Data)
0.038	Bagel, plain, unenriched w/ calcium propionate, onion, poppy, sesame (no cream cheese)
0.038	Chili powder
0.038	New England clam chowder, Campbell's Select (Missing Data)
0.038	Beets, raw
0.037	Pistachio nuts, dry roasted, no salt
0.037	Peanut butter, smooth, USDA Commodity
0.037	Banquest Hearty Ones Salisbury Steak Dinner w/ Gravy, Mashed Potatoes and Corn in Seasoned Sauce, frozen meal(Missing Data)
0.037	Almonds, USDA A256, A264
0.037	Whole wheat pita bread
0.037	Saffron (Missing Data)
0.037	Spaghetti, cooked, enriched w/out added salt, no sauce
0.036	Quinoa, cooked
0.036	Oregano, dried
0.036	Oats, unenriched, boiled, w/out salt
0.035	Cardamom (Missing Data)
0.035	Barley (hulled)
0.035	Hotdog, Oscar Mayer Wiener, beef frank (No Trans Fat Data)
0.034	Poppy seed
0.034	Flaxseed
0.034	Roll, hard, kaiser
0.034	Sage, ground

0.033	Popcorn, air-popped
0.033	Sunflower Seeds, hulled, dry roasted, no salt
0.033	White pita bread, enriched
0.033	Egg noodles, cooked, enriched
0.033	Thyme, dried
0.033	Peppers, sweet, red, raw
0.032	Chia seeds, dried (Missing Sugar and Vitamin Data)
0.032	Wheat dinner rolls
0.031	Ginger, ground
0.031	Cheerios, General Mills
0.031	Pretzels, hard, whole-wheat (Missing Sugar Data)
0.031	Corn, sweet, yellow, boiled, drained, no salt
0.030	Whole wheat bread, prepared from recipe
0.030	Beets, canned, drained solids
0.030	Cream of Wheat, instant, prepared with water and salt
0.029	Millet, cooked
0.029	Bran Flakes, single brand
0.029	Banquet chicken pot pie, frozen entrée (Missing Data)
0.029	White bread, commercially prepared (inlcudes soft crumbs)
0.028	Mushrooms, shiitake, cooked, no salt
0.028	White flour, white, all-purpose, enriched, bleached
0.028	Onion, raw
0.027	Pretzels, hard, plain, salted
0.027	Wheaties, General Mills
0.027	Potato, Russet, baked, flesh & skin
0.027	Potato, baked, flesh & skin, no salt
0.027	Cashews, dry roasted, no salt
0.027	Kellogg's Raisin Bran
0.027	Popcorn, microwave, 94% fat free
0.026	Potato, red, baked, flesh & skin
0.026	Avg. Nuts
0.026	Cantaloupe, raw
0.026	Bay leaf (Missing Data)
0.025	Matzo crackers, plain
0.025	Rosemarry, fresh (Missing Data)

0.025	Horseradish, prepared
0.024	Ramen noodle soup, chicken flavor, dry
0.024	Eggplant, boiled, drained, no salt
0.024	Pretzels, soft
0.024	Spaghetti squash, winter, boiled w/out salt, drained
0.024	Grits, corn, white, regular, quick, enriched, cooked with water, with salt
0.024	Parboiled rice, white, long-grain, enriched, cooked
0.024	Peaches, raw
0.023	Raspberries, raw
0.023	Walnuts, USDA A259, A257
0.023	Brown rice, long-grain, cooked
0.023	Carrots, raw, USDA A099
0.023	Allspice (Missing Data)
0.022	Sweet potato, baked in skin, no salt
0.022	Turmeric, ground
0.022	Butternut squash, winter, baked w/out salt, sugar or butter
0.022	Brazil nuts, dried, unblanched
0.021	Rice cakes, brown rice, plain
0.021	Instant Oatmeal, Quaker, apples & cinnamon prepared w/ boiling water
0.021	White rice, glutinous, cooked
0.020	White rice, long-grain, regular, cooked
0.020	Pomegranate, raw
0.020	Strawberries, raw
0.020	Sesame sticks, wheat-based, salted
0.020	Orange, raw, all commercial varieties
0.020	Post Honey Bunches of Oats w/ Almonds (Missing Data)
0.019	Potato flour
0.019	White rice, long-grain, pre-cooked or instant, prepared (Missing O3FA Data)
0.019	Cloves, ground
0.018	Ice cream, soft-serve, french vanilla (No Trans Fat Data)
0.018	Corn Flakes, Kellogg's
0.018	Ketchup
0.018	Rice Krispies, Kellogg's
0.017	Cream cheese (No Trans Fat Data)

0.017	Cherries, sweet, raw
0.017	Lucky Charms, General Mills
0.017	Peanut Butter Cap'n Crunch, Quaker
0.017	Ice creams, vanilla (No Trans Fat Data)
0.017	Honey Smacks, Kellogg's
0.017	Popcorn, regular butter flavor, microwave, made w/ partially hydrogenated oil (Missing Fats Data)
0.016	Mashed potatoes, home-prepared, whole milk & butter added
0.016	Lemon juice, raw
0.016	Papayas, raw
0.016	Cinnamon
0.016	Avg. Fruit
0.016	FritoLay Sun Chips, Multi-grain snack, original flavor
0.016	Candy bar, Snickers (King Size)
0.016	Tortilla chips, plain, white corn
0.015	Rosemary, dried (Missing Data)
0.015	Mace, ground (Missing Data)
0.015	Ritz Crackers, Nabisco (Missing Vitamin Data)
0.015	Tortilla chips, plain, yellow corn (Missing Vitamin Data)
0.014	Milk chocolate candies (No Trans Fat Data)
0.014	Golden Crisp, Post, Kraft
0.014	Cocoa Krispies, Kellogg's (No O3FA Data)
0.013	Granola bar, soft, uncoated, chocolate chip
0.013	Pecans, dry roasted, no salt
0.013	Honeycomb cereal, Post, Kraft (low data)
0.012	Avocado, raw, commercial varieties
0.012	Banana, raw
0.012	Blueberries, raw
0.012	Cinnamon Toast Crunch cereal, ready-to-eat, General Mills
0.012	McDonald's French Fries
0.012	Potato chips, plain, salted
0.012	Kellogg's Nutri-Grain Cereal Bars, fruit-filled
0.012	Frosted Flakes, Kellogg's
0.012	Corn chips, extruded, plain
0.011	Nutmeg, ground (Missing O3FA Data)

0.011	Pineapple, raw, all varieties
0.011	Cap'n Crunch, Quaker
0.011	Cap'n Crunch with Crunch Berries, Quaker
0.011	Macadamia nuts, dry roasted, with salt
0.011	Macadamia nuts, dry roasted, w/out salt
0.011	Apple Jacks, Kellogg's
0.011	Dark chocolate candies, 60-69% cacao solids (Missing Vitamin Data)
0.011	Grapes, red or green, European type such as Thompson seedless, raw
0.010	Raisins, seedless
0.010	Cheese-flavor puffs or twists, corn-based
0.010	Chocolate-flavored hazelnut spread (No Trans Fat Data)
0.010	Corn Pops, Kellogg's
0.009	Coconut meat, raw
0.009	McDonald's barbeque sauce
0.009	Cake, snack cakes, crème-filled, chocolate with frosting
0.009	Popcorn, caramel-coated without peanuts
0.009	Froot Loops, General Mills
0.008	Rice noodles, cooked (Missing Sugar & Unsaturated Fat Data)
0.008	Pineapple, canned, juice pack, drained
0.008	Cocoa Puffs, General Mills
0.007	Mangos, raw
0.007	Olives, pickled, canned or bottled, green
0.006	Grape Juice, canned or bottled, unsweetened
0.005	Apple, raw, with skin A343
0.005	Cheetos Crunchy cheese-flavored snacks (No O3, 6FA Data)
0.004	Banana chips
0.004	McDonald's spicy buffalo sauce
0.003	Apricot jam and preserves
0.003	Light mayo (salad dressing)
0.003	Margarine, industrial, non-dairy, cottonseed, soy oil (partially hydrogenated), for flaky pastries
0.002	Apple Juice, canned or bottled, unsweetened
0.001	Sprite
0.001	Mayonnaise, soybean oil, w/ salt (salad dressing)

0.001	Butter, salted (No Trans Fat Data)
0.001	Honey
0.001	Corn starch (Missing O3FA Data)

Vitamin A

Vitamin A, IU/SS	Food
527.420	Paprika
296.490	Chili powder
192.165	Sweet potato, baked in skin, no salt
167.055	Carrots, raw, USDA A099
136.223	Kale, boiled, drained, no salt
111.556	Butternut squash, winter, baked w/out salt, sugar or butter
104.817	Spinach, boiled, drained, no salt
101.830	Parsley, dried (Missing O3FA Data)
93.760	Basil, dried
87.110	Romaine or cos lettuce
80.670	Marjoram, dried
78.407	Avg. Spice
69.030	Oregano, dried
68.094	Avg. Herbs
64.022	Avg. Leafy Green Vegetables
61.850	Bay leaf (Missing Data)
61.240	Swiss chard, boiled, drained, no salt
59.000	Sage, ground
58.510	Cilantro, dried (No O3FA Data)
58.510	Dill weed, dried (Missing Data)
52.760	Basil, fresh
47.510	Thyme, fresh (Missing Data)
42.860	Margarine, industrial, non-dairy, cottonseed, soy oil (partially hydrogenated), for flaky pastries
42.488	Pak-choi, boiled, drained, no salt
42.000	Tarragon, dried (Missing Data)
40.540	Spearmint, fresh (Missing Data)
38.010	Thyme, dried
35.710	Margarine (vegetable oil spread, 70% fat, soybean & partially hydrogenated soybean, stick)
33.824	Cantaloupe, raw
32.990	Cinnamon Toast Crunch cereal, ready-to-eat, General Mills
31.315	Peppers, sweet, red, raw
31.280	Rosemary, dried (Missing Data)

29.240	Rosemarry, fresh (Missing Data)
28.880	Cheerios, General Mills
27.780	Golden Crisp, Post, Kraft
27.310	Apple Jacks, Kellogg's
25.860	Honeycomb cereal, Post, Kraft (low data)
25.000	Bran Flakes, single brand
24.991	Butter, salted (No Trans Fat Data)
24.190	Post Honey Bunches of Oats w/ Almonds (Missing Data)
20.996	Peas, frozen, boiled, drained, no salt
20.270	Kellogg's Nutri-Grain Cereal Bars, fruit-filled
19.610	Frosted Flakes, Kellogg's
18.890	Rice Krispies, Kellogg's
18.850	Honey Smacks, Kellogg's
18.600	Lucky Charms, General Mills
18.585	Avg. Vegetables
17.910	Corn Flakes, Kellogg's
16.670	Wheaties, General Mills
16.400	Cocoa Krispies, Kellogg's (No O3FA Data)
16.140	Corn Pops, Kellogg's
16.100	Froot Loops, General Mills
15.479	Broccoli, boiled, drained, no salt
14.720	Kellogg's Raisin Bran
12.700	Cumin seed
12.647	Cream cheese (No Trans Fat Data)
11.172	Zucchini, summer squash, w/ skin, boiled w/out salt, drained
11.070	Velveeta cheese, Kraft, pasteurized spread (Missing Data)
10.936	Papayas, raw
10.280	McDonald's spicy buffalo sauce
10.023	Cheddar cheese (No Trans Fat Data)
9.860	Curry powder
9.610	American cheese, pasteurized, w/out disodium phosphate (No Trans Fat Data)
9.329	Ketchup
8.803	Provolone cheese (No Trans Fat Data)
8.329	Tomatoes, raw, red, ripe
8.303	Swiss Cheese (No Trans Fat Data)

8.072	Avg. Cheese
8.000	Mace, ground (Missing Data)
7.730	Cream of Wheat, instant, prepared with water and salt
7.670	Acerola (West Indian cherry), raw (Missing Sugar and Vitamin Data)
7.648	Mangos, raw
7.630	Blue Cheese (No Trans Fat Data)
7.560	Asparagus, raw
7.181	Instant Oatmeal, Quaker, apples & cinnamon prepared w/ boiling water
7.000	Snap (green string) beans, boiled, drained, no salt
6.919	Banquet chicken pot pie, frozen entrée (Missing Data)
6.759	Mozzarella cheese, whole milk (No Trans Fat Data)
5.890	Ice cream, soft-serve, french vanilla (No Trans Fat Data)
5.700	Clams, mixed species, cooked in moist heat
5.500	Salsa, USDA Commodity (Missing Sugar and Vitamin Data)
5.400	Allspice (Missing Data)
5.300	Cloves, ground
5.300	Saffron (Missing Data)
5.260	Egg, whole, cooked, scrambled
5.020	Iceberg lettuce
4.810	Mozzarella cheese, part skim (No Trans Fat Data)
4.579	Milk, nonfat, Ca fortified
4.450	Ricotta cheese, whole milk (No Trans Fat Data)
4.429	Avg. Fruit
4.420	Parmesan cheese, grated (No Trans Fat Data)
4.331	Tomato sauce, canned
4.210	Ice creams, vanilla (No Trans Fat Data)
3.930	Olives, pickled, canned or bottled, green
3.698	Peppers, sweet, green, raw
3.630	Caraway seed
3.583	Slice of pizza, fast food, pizza chain, 14", cheese topping, regular crust (No Trans Fat Data)
3.330	Culver's shrimp cocktail sauce (Missing Vitamin Data)
3.257	Peaches, raw
3.130	Salsa, Campbell Pace, Thick & Chunky (Missing Vitamin Data)
3.110	Anise seed (Missing Sugar, Vitamin, O3FA data)

3.029	Lima beans, immature, boiled, drained, no salt
2.990	Black pepper
2.950	Cinnamon
2.883	Avg. Beans & Lentils
2.800	Mayonnaise, soybean oil, w/ salt (salad dressing)
2.640	Popcorn, microwave, 94% fat free
2.628	Corn, sweet, yellow, boiled, drained, no salt
2.618	Pistachio nuts, dry roasted, no salt
2.520	Popcorn, regular butter flavor, microwave, made w/ partially hydrogenated oil (Missing Fats Data)
2.500	Beef sticks, smoked (No Trans Fat Data)
2.370	McDonald's barbeque sauce
2.300	Orange, raw, all commercial varieties
2.250	Shrimp, mixed species, cooked in moist heat
2.200	Light mayo (salad dressing)
2.050	Apricot jam and preserves
2.041	Milk, nonfat, added Vit A
2.008	Chicken noodle soup prepared with equal volume water
1.960	Popcorn, air-popped
1.959	Milk, lowfat, 1%, added Vit A
1.952	Milk chocolate candies (No Trans Fat Data)
1.889	Milk, reduced fat, 2%, added Vit A
1.839	Weight Watchers Smart Ones Chicken Enchiladas Suiza, Sour Cream w/ Cheese frozen entrée (Missing Data)
1.832	Pickles, cucumber, dill or kosher dill
1.800	Oysters, eastern, wild, cooked, moist heat
1.690	Candy bar, Snickers (King Size)
1.620	Hot Sauce (ready-to-serve, sauce, pepper or hot)
1.510	Peanut Butter Cap'n Crunch, Quaker
1.470	Cap'n Crunch, Quaker
1.458	Avocado, raw, commercial varieties
1.440	Cap'n Crunch with Crunch Berries, Quaker
1.400	Pecans, dry roasted, no salt
1.368	Swordfish, cooked in dry heat
1.350	Fennel seed (Missing Vitamin & O3FA Data)
1.300	Mashed potatoes, home-prepared, whole milk & butter added
1.270	Cheese-flavor puffs or twists, corn-based

1.153	Red snapper, cooked, dry heat
1.143	Avg. Seafood
1.130	Whiting, mixed species, cooked in dry heat
1.097	Spaghetti squash, winter, boiled w/out salt, drained
1.050	Cucumber, raw w/ peel
1.020	Milk, whole, 3.25% milkfat
1.020	Nutmeg, ground (Missing O3FA Data)
1.000	Scallops (bay & sea), steamed
1.000	Oysters, eastern, wild, raw
0.869	Lobster, northern, cooked in moist heat
0.849	Turkey, stuffing, mashed potatoes w/ gravy, assorted vegetables, frozen, microwaved
0.830	Banana chips
0.800	Cabbage, boiled, drained, no salt
0.750	Bologna, chicken, pork, beef
0.720	Kraft macaroni & cheese dinner, original, unprepared (Missing Data)
0.711	Mustard, prepared, yellow
0.660	Grapes, red or green, European type such as Thompson seedless, raw
0.640	Cherries, sweet, raw
0.640	Banana, raw
0.620	Mustard seed, yellow
0.620	Pumpkin/Squash Seeds, dry roasted, no salt (Missing Vitamin & Se Data)
0.600	Fenugreek seed (Missing Vitamin & O3, 6FA Data)
0.580	Pineapple, raw, all varieties
0.560	Tuna fish, light, canned in water without salt, drained solids
0.540	Blueberries, raw
0.538	Apple, raw, with skin A343
0.520	Celery seed
0.510	Yogurt, regular low-fat, plain, 12 g protein per 8 oz
0.500	Pineapple, canned, juice pack, drained
0.500	Dark chocolate candies, 60-69% cacao solids (Missing Vitamin Data)
0.500	Crayfish, mixed species, farmed, cooked in moist heat
0.480	Avg. Nuts
0.440	Salmon, Atlantic, wild, cooked in dry heat

0.430	Flounder (sole), cooked in dry heat
0.420	Pastrami luncheon meat, beef, cured (No Trans Fat Data)
0.412	Ginger, ground
0.410	Cottage cheese, 1% milkfat (No Trans Fat Data)
0.400	Pork-skins, plain
0.400	Anchovies, European, canned in oil, drained solids
0.390	Bologna, lebanon, beef (No O3FA Data)
0.370	Eggplant, boiled, drained, no salt
0.370	Bacon (pork), cured, cooked, pan-fried
0.330	Beets, raw
0.330	Raspberries, raw
0.320	Sausage, Italian, pork, cooked (No Trans Fat Data)
0.280	Cocoa Puffs, General Mills
0.270	Chick peas (garbanzo, bengal gram), mature seeds, boiled, no salt
0.240	Beets, canned, drained solids
0.220	Barley (hulled)
0.213	Avg. Cased Meat
0.210	Egg noodles, cooked, enriched
0.210	Chick peas (garbanzo, bengal gram), mature seeds, canned
0.210	Chicken, broilers or fryers, breast, meat only (no skin), roasted
0.200	Lemon juice, raw
0.200	Walnuts, USDA A259, A257
0.200	Chamomile Tea (No O3FA & O6FA Data)
0.190	Tuna fish, white, canned in water without salt, drained solids
0.133	Greek style yogurt 150g=2/3 cup (Missing Data)
0.130	Cauliflower, raw
0.120	Strawberries, raw
0.110	Rye
0.100	Potato, baked, flesh & skin, no salt
0.100	Potato, red, baked, flesh & skin
0.100	Potato, Russet, baked, flesh & skin
0.090	Soybeans green, boiled, drained, no salt
0.090	Whole wheat flour
0.090	Sunflower Seeds, hulled, dry roasted, no salt
0.090	Garlic, raw
0.080	Popcorn, caramel-coated without peanuts

0.080	Cranberry juice cocktail, bottled
0.080	Grape Juice, canned or bottled, unsweetened
0.080	Lentils, mature seeds, boiled, no salt
0.070	Radishes, raw
0.053	Avg. Lean Meat
0.050	Quinoa, cooked
0.050	Sesame sticks, wheat-based, salted
0.050	Hummus, home prepared
0.040	Black beans, mature seeds, canned
0.030	Whole wheat bread, commecially prepared
0.030	Whole wheat bread, prepared from recipe
0.030	Tortilla chips, plain, white corn
0.030	Chocolate-flavored hazelnut spread (No Trans Fat Data)
0.030	Millet, cooked
0.030	Wild rice, cooked
0.020	Onion, raw
0.020	Cake, snack cakes, crème-filled, chocolate with frosting
0.020	Horseradish, prepared
0.010	Ramen noodle soup, chicken flavor, dry
0.010	Apple Juice, canned or bottled, unsweetened
0.010	Almonds, USDA A256, A264

Vitamin C

Vitamin C, mg/SS	Food
16.770	Acerola (West Indian cherry), raw (Missing Sugar and Vitamin Data)
5.670	Cilantro, dried (No O3FA Data)
1.800	Culver's shrimp cocktail sauce (Missing Vitamin Data)
1.600	Thyme, fresh (Missing Data)
1.275	Peppers, sweet, red, raw
1.220	Parsley, dried (Missing O3FA Data)
0.808	Cloves, ground
0.808	Saffron (Missing Data)
0.805	Peppers, sweet, green, raw
0.748	Hot Sauce (ready-to-serve, sauce, pepper or hot)
0.711	Paprika
0.650	Broccoli, boiled, drained, no salt
0.641	Chili powder
0.618	Papayas, raw
0.612	Basil, dried
0.612	Rosemary, dried (Missing Data)
0.594	Apple Jacks, Kellogg's
0.588	Strawberries, raw
0.544	Orange, raw, all commercial varieties
0.514	Marjoram, dried
0.500	Oregano, dried
0.500	Thyme, dried
0.500	Tarragon, dried (Missing Data)
0.500	Dill weed, dried (Missing Data)
0.490	Avg. Herbs
0.484	Cocoa Krispies, Kellogg's (No O3FA Data)
0.478	Pineapple, raw, all varieties
0.470	Froot Loops, General Mills
0.465	Bay leaf (Missing Data)
0.464	Cauliflower, raw
0.462	Apple, raw, with skin A343
0.459	Lemon juice, raw
0.423	Cranberry juice cocktail, bottled

0.410	Kale, boiled, drained, no salt
0.392	Allspice (Missing Data)
0.375	Cabbage, boiled, drained, no salt
0.367	Cantaloupe, raw
0.324	Sage, ground
0.316	Avg. Leafy Green Vegetables
0.312	Garlic, raw
0.297	Avg. Spice
0.295	Avg. Fruit
0.280	Avg. Vegetables
0.278	Rice Krispies, Kellogg's
0.277	Mangos, raw
0.267	Frosted Flakes, Kellogg's
0.262	Raspberries, raw
0.260	Pak-choi, boiled, drained, no salt
0.259	Turmeric, ground
0.249	Horseradish, prepared
0.244	Cheerios, General Mills
0.240	Romaine or cos lettuce
0.235	Cinnamon Toast Crunch cereal, ready-to-eat, General Mills
0.233	Lucky Charms, General Mills
0.226	Honey Smacks, Kellogg's
0.221	Clams, mixed species, cooked in moist heat
0.220	Corn Flakes, Kellogg's
0.218	Rosemarry, fresh (Missing Data)
0.210	Caraway seed
0.210	Black pepper
0.210	Anise seed (Missing Sugar, Vitamin, O3FA data)
0.210	Cardamom (Missing Data)
0.210	Mace, ground (Missing Data)
0.210	Coriander seed (Missing Data)
0.210	Fennel seed (Missing Vitamin & O3FA Data)
0.200	Wheaties, General Mills
0.200	Cocoa Puffs, General Mills
0.196	Sweet potato, baked in skin, no salt
0.194	Corn Pops, Kellogg's

0.186	Potato chips, plain, salted
0.180	Swiss chard, boiled, drained, no salt
0.180	Basil, fresh
0.171	Celery seed
0.171	Strawberry Jam, Hardee's condiment (Missing Data)
0.158	Bologna, chicken, pork, beef
0.151	Butternut squash, winter, baked w/out salt, sugar or butter
0.151	Ketchup
0.148	Radishes, raw
0.133	Spearmint, fresh (Missing Data)
0.129	Potato, Russet, baked, flesh & skin
0.127	Tomatoes, raw, red, ripe
0.126	Potato, red, baked, flesh & skin
0.114	Curry powder
0.108	Grapes, red or green, European type such as Thompson seedless, raw
0.102	Pomegranate, raw
0.101	Lima beans, immature, boiled, drained, no salt
0.100	Avocado, raw, commercial varieties
0.099	Peas, frozen, boiled, drained, no salt
0.098	Spinach, boiled, drained, no salt
0.097	Blueberries, raw
0.097	Snap (green string) beans, boiled, drained, no salt
0.096	Potato, baked, flesh & skin, no salt
0.094	Pineapple, canned, juice pack, drained
0.088	Apricot jam and preserves
0.087	Banana, raw
0.079	Hummus, home prepared
0.077	Cumin seed
0.074	Onion, raw
0.073	McDonald's French Fries
0.070	Cherries, sweet, raw
0.070	Tomato sauce, canned
0.068	Beef sticks, smoked (No Trans Fat Data)
0.066	Peaches, raw
0.063	Banana chips
0.062	Corn, sweet, yellow, boiled, drained, no salt

0.061	Edamame beans, frozen, prepared
0.060	Oysters, eastern, wild, cooked, moist heat
0.060	Mashed potatoes, home-prepared, whole milk & butter added
0.059	Carrots, raw, USDA A099
0.056	Asparagus, raw
0.049	Beets, raw
0.046	Zucchini, summer squash, w/ skin, boiled w/out salt, drained
0.046	Soybeans (aka soy nuts) mature, dry roasted (Missing Sugar and Vitamin Data)
0.044	Avg. Beans & Lentils
0.041	Beets, canned, drained solids
0.040	Salsa, USDA Commodity (Missing Sugar and Vitamin Data)
0.040	Mushrooms, boiled, drained, no salt
0.038	Potato flour
0.038	Cinnamon
0.038	Chick peas (garbanzo, bengal gram), mature seeds, canned
0.037	Oysters, eastern, wild, raw
0.035	Spaghetti squash, winter, boiled w/out salt, drained
0.033	Coconut meat, raw
0.030	Mustard seed, yellow
0.030	Fenugreek seed (Missing Vitamin & O3, 6FA Data)
0.030	Nutmeg, ground (Missing O3FA Data)
0.028	Iceberg lettuce
0.028	Cucumber, raw w/ peel
0.027	Black beans, mature seeds, canned
0.024	Avg. Cased Meat
0.023	Raisins, seedless
0.023	Pistachio nuts, dry roasted, no salt
0.022	Shrimp, mixed species, cooked in moist heat
0.021	Avg. Seafood
0.020	Ginger, ground
0.019	Cake, snack cakes, crème-filled, chocolate with frosting
0.017	Soybeans green, boiled, drained, no salt
0.016	Red snapper, cooked, dry heat
0.015	Lentils, mature seeds, boiled, no salt
0.015	Weight Watchers Smart Ones Chicken Enchiladas Suiza, Sour Cream w/ Cheese frozen entrée (Missing Data)

0.015	Mustard, prepared, yellow
0.014	Sunflower Seeds, hulled, dry roasted, no salt
0.013	Eggplant, boiled, drained, no salt
0.013	Walnuts, USDA A259, A257
0.013	Chick peas (garbanzo, bengal gram), mature seeds, boiled, no salt
0.012	Kidney beans, red, boiled, no salt, mature seeds
0.011	Swordfish, cooked in dry heat
0.010	Milk, nonfat, Ca fortified
0.010	Poppy seed
0.010	Pretzels, hard, whole-wheat (Missing Sugar Data)
0.009	Apple Juice, canned or bottled, unsweetened
0.009	Bologna, lebanon, beef (No O3FA Data)
0.009	Spam, Hormel (Missing Data)
0.008	Pinto beans, boiled, no salt, mature
0.008	Yogurt, regular low-fat, plain, 12 g protein per 8 oz
0.008	Turkey, stuffing, mashed potatoes w/ gravy, assorted vegetables, frozen, microwaved
0.008	Ice cream, soft-serve, french vanilla (No Trans Fat Data)
0.008	Avg. Nuts
0.008	Pickles, cucumber, dill or kosher dill
0.007	Pecans, dry roasted, no salt
0.007	Pepperoni, pork, beef
0.007	Macadamia nuts, dry roasted, with salt
0.007	Macadamia nuts, dry roasted, w/out salt
0.007	Brazil nuts, dried, unblanched
0.006	Flaxseed
0.006	Ice creams, vanilla (No Trans Fat Data)
0.005	Candy bar, Snickers (King Size)
0.005	Honey
0.005	Pork-skins, plain
0.005	Crayfish, mixed species, farmed, cooked in moist heat
0.005	Kraft macaroni & cheese dinner, original, unprepared (Missing Data)
0.004	Margarine, industrial, non-dairy, cottonseed, soy oil (partially hydrogenated), for flaky pastries
0.003	Pastrami luncheon meat, beef, cured (No Trans Fat Data)
0.003	Pumpkin/Squash Seeds, dry roasted, no salt (Missing Vitamin & Se Data)

0.003	Mushrooms, shiitake, cooked, no salt
0.002	Milk, reduced fat, 2%, added Vit A
0.002	Instant Oatmeal, Quaker, apples & cinnamon prepared w/ boiling water
0.002	Egg, whole, cooked, scrambled
0.002	Velveeta cheese, Kraft, pasteurized spread (Missing Data)
0.001	Grape Juice, canned or bottled, unsweetened
0.001	Cap'n Crunch with Crunch Berries, Quaker
0.001	Sausage, Italian, pork, cooked (No Trans Fat Data)
0.001	Post Honey Bunches of Oats w/ Almonds (Missing Data)

Vitamin D

Vitamin D, IU/SS	Food
3.202	Oysters, eastern, wild, raw
1.620	Corn Pops, Kellogg's
1.520	Corn Flakes, Kellogg's
1.480	Lucky Charms, General Mills
1.480	Honey Smacks, Kellogg's
1.480	Golden Crisp, Post, Kraft
1.380	Honeycomb cereal, Post, Kraft (low data)
1.330	Cheerios, General Mills
1.330	Bran Flakes, single brand
1.330	Wheaties, General Mills
1.330	Cinnamon Toast Crunch cereal, ready-to-eat, General Mills
1.300	Cocoa Krispies, Kellogg's (No O3FA Data)
1.290	Frosted Flakes, Kellogg's
1.290	Post Honey Bunches of Oats w/ Almonds (Missing Data)
1.270	Apple Jacks, Kellogg's
1.250	Froot Loops, General Mills
1.240	Rice Krispies, Kellogg's
0.680	Kellogg's Raisin Bran
0.559	Butter, salted (No Trans Fat Data)
0.520	Milk, lowfat, 1%, added Vit A
0.480	Salami, cooked, beef (No Trans Fat Data)
0.440	Swiss Cheese (No Trans Fat Data)
0.430	Milk, reduced fat, 2%, added Vit A
0.408	Milk, nonfat, added Vit A
0.400	Milk, whole, 3.25% milkfat
0.340	Egg, whole, cooked, scrambled
0.240	Hotdog, Oscar Mayer Wiener, beef frank (No Trans Fat Data)
0.210	Mushrooms, boiled, drained, no salt
0.210	Mushrooms, canned, drained solids
0.187	Avg. Cheese
0.162	Avg. Cased Meat
0.120	Cheddar cheese (No Trans Fat Data)
0.090	Pepperoni, pork, beef

| 0.080 | Mashed potatoes, home-prepared, whole milk & butter added |
| 0.010 | Cheese-flavor puffs or twists, corn-based |

Vitamin E

Vitamin E, mg/SS	Food
0.411	Sunflower oil (vegetable oil) (Missing Trans Fat & Phytosterol Data)
0.353	Cottonseed (vegetable oil), salad or cooking (Missing Trans Fat Data)
0.341	Safflower oil (vegetable oil), salad or cooking, linoleic, (over 70%) (No Trans Fat or O3FA Data)
0.298	Paprika
0.291	Chili powder
0.288	Grapeseed oil (vegetable oil) (Missing Trans Fat Data)
0.262	Almonds, USDA A256, A264
0.261	Sunflower Seeds, hulled, dry roasted, no salt
0.220	Curry powder
0.189	Oregano, dried
0.175	Canola oil (vegetable oil), low erucic acid rapeseed oil
0.159	Palm oil (Missing Trans Fat Data)
0.156	Peanut oil, salad or cooking (No Trans Fat or O3FA Data)
0.144	Olive oil (Missing Trans Fat Data)
0.143	Corn oil (vegetable oil), industrial and retail, all purpose salad or cooking
0.096	Avg. Spice
0.086	Avg. Herbs
0.085	Cloves, ground
0.082	Soybean oil, salad or cooking (Missing Phytosterol Data)
0.081	Shortening, vegetable, industrial, soy (partially hydrogenated), all purpose
0.075	Basil, dried
0.075	Sage, ground
0.075	Thyme, dried
0.073	Avg. Nuts
0.070	FritoLay Sun Chips, Multi-grain snack, original flavor
0.069	Peanuts, dry roasted, no salt, all types
0.069	Parsley, dried (Missing O3FA Data)
0.067	Potato chips, plain, salted
0.059	Peanut butter, smooth, USDA Commodity
0.057	Brazil nuts, dried, unblanched
0.056	Margarine (vegetable oil spread, 70% fat, soybean & partially hydrogenated soybean, stick)

0.052	Mayonnaise, soybean oil, w/ salt (salad dressing)
0.050	Chocolate-flavored hazelnut spread (No Trans Fat Data)
0.050	Ginger, ground
0.047	Cheese-flavor puffs or twists, corn-based
0.046	Margarine, industrial, non-dairy, cottonseed, soy oil (partially hydrogenated), for flaky pastries
0.043	Tortilla chips, plain, white corn
0.038	Olives, pickled, canned or bottled, green
0.038	Sesame sticks, wheat-based, salted
0.035	Ritz Crackers, Nabisco (Missing Vitamin Data)
0.033	Anchovies, European, canned in oil, drained solids
0.033	Cumin seed
0.031	Light mayo (salad dressing)
0.031	Turmeric, ground
0.029	Mustard seed, yellow
0.027	McDonald's spicy buffalo sauce
0.025	Caraway seed
0.023	Butter, salted (No Trans Fat Data)
0.023	Cinnamon
0.023	Cheetos Crunchy cheese-flavored snacks (No O3, 6FA Data)
0.021	Avocado, raw, commercial varieties
0.021	Spinach, boiled, drained, no salt
0.020	Cinnamon Toast Crunch cereal, ready-to-eat, General Mills
0.020	Pistachio nuts, dry roasted, no salt
0.019	Swiss chard, boiled, drained, no salt
0.018	Poppy seed
0.018	Popcorn, regular butter flavor, microwave, made w/ partially hydrogenated oil (Missing Fats Data)
0.017	Marjoram, dried
0.016	Peppers, sweet, red, raw
0.015	Candy bar, Snickers (King Size)
0.015	Scallops (bay & sea), steamed
0.015	Ramen noodle soup, chicken flavor, dry
0.015	Broccoli, boiled, drained, no salt
0.015	Ketchup
0.014	Avg. Seafood
0.014	Tomato sauce, canned

0.014	Sesame oil (Missing Trans Fat Data)
0.014	Shrimp, mixed species, cooked in moist heat
0.014	Corn chips, extruded, plain
0.013	Rye
0.013	Pecans, dry roasted, no salt
0.013	Butternut squash, winter, baked w/out salt, sugar or butter
0.012	Rice cakes, brown rice, plain
0.012	Popcorn, caramel-coated without peanuts
0.012	Wheaties, General Mills
0.011	Asparagus, raw
0.011	Cake, snack cakes, crème-filled, chocolate with frosting
0.011	McDonald's barbeque sauce
0.011	Egg, whole, cooked, scrambled
0.011	Celery seed
0.011	Mangos, raw
0.010	Lobster, northern, cooked in moist heat
0.010	Cilantro, dried (No O3FA Data)
0.009	Cashews, dry roasted, no salt
0.009	Avg. Leafy Green Vegetables
0.009	Pinto beans, boiled, no salt, mature
0.009	Bran Flakes, single brand
0.009	Raspberries, raw
0.009	Slice of pizza, fast food, pizza chain, 14", cheese topping, regular crust (No Trans Fat Data)
0.008	Oysters, eastern, wild, raw
0.008	Kale, boiled, drained, no salt
0.008	Whole wheat flour
0.008	Whole wheat bread, prepared from recipe
0.008	Cocoa Puffs, General Mills
0.008	Tilapia, cooked in dry heat
0.008	Basil, fresh
0.008	Shortening, industrial, soy (partially hydrogenated) for baking & confections (Missing O3FA Data)
0.008	Vegetable shortening, household, composite
0.007	Peaches, raw
0.007	Hummus, home prepared
0.007	Papayas, raw

0.007	Edamame beans, frozen, prepared
0.007	Sweet potato, baked in skin, no salt
0.007	Cheerios, General Mills
0.007	Kellogg's Raisin Bran
0.007	Cap'n Crunch, Quaker
0.007	Peanut Butter Cap'n Crunch, Quaker
0.007	Black pepper
0.007	Walnuts, USDA A259, A257
0.006	Quinoa, cooked
0.006	Cream cheese (No Trans Fat Data)
0.006	Flounder (sole), cooked in dry heat
0.006	Carrots, raw, USDA A099
0.006	Macadamia nuts, dry roasted, with salt
0.006	Macadamia nuts, dry roasted, w/out salt
0.006	Pomegranate, raw
0.006	Blueberries, raw
0.006	Whole wheat pita bread
0.006	Kellogg's Nutri-Grain Cereal Bars, fruit-filled
0.006	Cap'n Crunch with Crunch Berries, Quaker
0.006	Ice cream, soft-serve, french vanilla (No Trans Fat Data)
0.006	Bologna, lebanon, beef (No O3FA Data)
0.006	Lard (No Trans Fat Data)
0.006	Pretzels, soft
0.006	Avg. Vegetables
0.005	Barley (hulled)
0.005	Tomatoes, raw, red, ripe
0.005	Milk chocolate candies (No Trans Fat Data)
0.005	Whole wheat bread, commecially prepared
0.005	Pork-skins, plain
0.005	Honey Smacks, Kellogg's
0.005	Hamburger patty, 80/20 ground chuck beef, broiled
0.005	Snap (green string) beans, boiled, drained, no salt
0.004	Avg. Fruit
0.004	Peppers, sweet, green, raw
0.004	Eggplant, boiled, drained, no salt
0.004	Roll, hard, kaiser

0.004	Wheat dinner rolls
0.004	Pretzels, hard, plain, salted
0.004	Popcorn, microwave, 94% fat free
0.004	Beef, eye of round, separable lean only, trimmed to 0" fat, all grades, roasted [cube steak]
0.004	Swiss Cheese (No Trans Fat Data)
0.004	Chick peas (garbanzo, bengal gram), mature seeds, boiled, no salt
0.004	Mustard, prepared, yellow
0.003	Soybeans green, boiled, drained, no salt
0.003	Avg. Cheese
0.003	Cheddar cheese (No Trans Fat Data)
0.003	Flaxseed
0.003	White pita bread, enriched
0.003	Popcorn, air-popped
0.003	Granola bar, soft, uncoated, chocolate chip
0.003	Lucky Charms, General Mills
0.003	Ice creams, vanilla (No Trans Fat Data)
0.003	American cheese, pasteurized, w/out disodium phosphate (No Trans Fat Data)
0.003	Parmesan cheese, grated (No Trans Fat Data)
0.003	Blue Cheese (No Trans Fat Data)
0.003	Ground turkey, cooked
0.003	Bacon (pork), cured, cooked, pan-fried
0.003	Whiting, mixed species, cooked in dry heat
0.003	Bologna, chicken, pork, beef
0.003	Sausage, Italian, pork, cooked (No Trans Fat Data)
0.003	Cocoa Krispies, Kellogg's (No O3FA Data)
0.003	Avg. Beans & Lentils
0.003	Chicken, broilers or fryers, breast, meat only (no skin), roasted
0.003	Strawberries, raw
0.003	Coconut meat, raw
0.003	Potato flour
0.002	Wild rice, cooked
0.002	Cranberry juice cocktail, bottled
0.002	Turkey, stuffing, mashed potatoes w/ gravy, assorted vegetables, frozen, microwaved
0.002	Provolone cheese (No Trans Fat Data)

0.002	Avg. Lean Meat
0.002	Iceberg lettuce
0.002	White bread, commercially prepared (inlcudes soft crumbs)
0.002	Banana chips
0.002	Salami, cooked, beef (No Trans Fat Data)
0.002	Corned beef luncheon meat, beef, cured, canned (No Trans Fat Data)
0.002	Grapes, red or green, European type such as Thompson seedless, raw
0.002	Egg noodles, cooked, enriched
0.002	Apple, raw, with skin A343
0.002	Mozzarella cheese, whole milk (No Trans Fat Data)
0.002	Orange, raw, all commercial varieties
0.002	Lemon juice, raw
0.002	Avg. Cased Meat
0.001	Mashed potatoes, home-prepared, whole milk & butter added
0.001	Spaghetti squash, winter, boiled w/out salt, drained
0.001	Raisins, seedless
0.001	Pak-choi, boiled, drained, no salt
0.001	Lima beans, immature, boiled, drained, no salt
0.001	Zucchini, summer squash, w/ skin, boiled w/out salt, drained
0.001	Lentils, mature seeds, boiled, no salt
0.001	Cauliflower, raw
0.001	Romaine or cos lettuce
0.001	Cabbage, boiled, drained, no salt
0.001	Matzo crackers, plain
0.001	Apricot jam and preserves
0.001	Hot Sauce (ready-to-serve, sauce, pepper or hot)
0.001	Corn Flakes, Kellogg's
0.001	Rice Krispies, Kellogg's
0.001	Froot Loops, General Mills
0.001	Apple Jacks, Kellogg's
0.001	Corn Pops, Kellogg's
0.001	Frosted Flakes, Kellogg's
0.001	Ricotta cheese, whole milk (No Trans Fat Data)
0.001	Mozzarella cheese, part skim (No Trans Fat Data)
0.001	Turkey, fryer-roaster, breast meat only, roasted
0.001	Pork tenderloin lean, roasted, URMIS 3358

0.001	Pastrami luncheon meat, beef, cured (No Trans Fat Data)
0.001	Cantaloupe, raw
0.001	Coconut oil (Missing Trans Fat & O3FA Data)
0.001	Oats, unenriched, boiled, w/out salt
0.001	White flour, white, all-purpose, enriched, bleached
0.001	Banana, raw
0.001	Garlic, raw
0.001	Beets, raw
0.001	Cherries, sweet, raw
0.001	Spaghetti, cooked, enriched w/out added salt, no sauce
0.001	Instant Oatmeal, Quaker, apples & cinnamon prepared w/ boiling water
0.001	Pickles, cucumber, dill or kosher dill
0.001	White rice, long-grain, regular, cooked
0.001	Corn, sweet, yellow, boiled, drained, no salt
0.001	White rice, glutinous, cooked
0.001	Kidney beans, red, boiled, no salt, mature seeds
0.001	Brown rice, long-grain, cooked

Vitamin K

Vitamin K, ug/SS	Food
17.150	Basil, dried
17.150	Sage, ground
17.150	Thyme, dried
13.600	Cilantro, dried (No O3FA Data)
13.600	Parsley, dried (Missing O3FA Data)
12.778	Avg. Herbs
8.169	Kale, boiled, drained, no salt
6.220	Marjoram, dried
6.220	Oregano, dried
4.939	Spinach, boiled, drained, no salt
4.150	Basil, fresh
3.274	Swiss chard, boiled, drained, no salt
2.893	Avg. Leafy Green Vegetables
1.839	Soybean oil, salad or cooking (Missing Phytosterol Data)
1.640	Black pepper
1.420	Cloves, ground
1.411	Broccoli, boiled, drained, no salt
1.090	Cabbage, boiled, drained, no salt
1.060	Chili powder
1.060	Margarine, industrial, non-dairy, cottonseed, soy oil (partially hydrogenated), for flaky pastries
1.030	Romaine or cos lettuce
0.998	Curry powder
0.803	Paprika
0.711	Canola oil (vegetable oil), low erucic acid rapeseed oil
0.602	Olive oil (Missing Trans Fat Data)
0.589	Avg. Spice
0.532	Vegetable shortening, household, composite
0.500	Ritz Crackers, Nabisco (Missing Vitamin Data)
0.430	Shortening, industrial, soy (partially hydrogenated) for baking & confections (Missing O3FA Data)
0.422	Mayonnaise, soybean oil, w/ salt (salad dressing)
0.416	Asparagus, raw
0.390	Pickles, cucumber, dill or kosher dill

0.370	Soybeans (aka soy nuts) mature, dry roasted (Missing Sugar and Vitamin Data)
0.347	Cashews, dry roasted, no salt
0.340	Pak-choi, boiled, drained, no salt
0.312	Cinnamon
0.267	Edamame beans, frozen, prepared
0.247	Cottonseed (vegetable oil), salad or cooking (Missing Trans Fat Data)
0.247	Shortening, vegetable, industrial, soy (partially hydrogenated), all purpose
0.247	Light mayo (salad dressing)
0.241	Iceberg lettuce
0.240	Peas, frozen, boiled, drained, no salt
0.221	Potato chips, plain, salted
0.210	Avocado, raw, commercial varieties
0.209	Tortilla chips, plain, white corn
0.193	Blueberries, raw
0.192	Soybeans green, boiled, drained, no salt
0.164	Cucumber, raw w/ peel
0.164	Pomegranate, raw
0.164	Granola bar, soft, uncoated, chocolate chip
0.160	Cauliflower, raw
0.160	Snap (green string) beans, boiled, drained, no salt
0.146	Grapes, red or green, European type such as Thompson seedless, raw
0.136	Sesame oil (Missing Trans Fat Data)
0.134	Turmeric, ground
0.132	Carrots, raw, USDA A099
0.132	Pistachio nuts, dry roasted, no salt
0.129	Kellogg's Nutri-Grain Cereal Bars, fruit-filled
0.125	Popcorn, caramel-coated without peanuts
0.121	Anchovies, European, canned in oil, drained solids
0.115	Turkey, stuffing, mashed potatoes w/ gravy, assorted vegetables, frozen, microwaved
0.112	Avg. Vegetables
0.106	Cake, snack cakes, crème-filled, chocolate with frosting
0.100	Avg. Beans & Lentils
0.094	Whole wheat bread, prepared from recipe

0.084	Kidney beans, red, boiled, no salt, mature seeds
0.080	Palm oil (Missing Trans Fat Data)
0.080	Sesame sticks, wheat-based, salted
0.079	Tomatoes, raw, red, ripe
0.078	Raspberries, raw
0.078	Whole wheat bread, commecially prepared
0.078	Cinnamon Toast Crunch cereal, ready-to-eat, General Mills
0.074	Peppers, sweet, green, raw
0.072	Dark chocolate candies, 60-69% cacao solids (Missing Vitamin Data)
0.071	Safflower oil (vegetable oil), salad or cooking, linoleic, (over 70%) (No Trans Fat or O3FA Data)
0.070	Butter, salted (No Trans Fat Data)
0.067	Slice of pizza, fast food, pizza chain, 14", cheese topping, regular crust (No Trans Fat Data)
0.063	Corn chips, extruded, plain
0.062	Lima beans, immature, boiled, drained, no salt
0.059	Avg. Nuts
0.059	Rye
0.058	Pepperoni, pork, beef
0.057	Milk chocolate candies (No Trans Fat Data)
0.056	Avg. Fruit
0.054	Sunflower oil (vegetable oil) (Missing Trans Fat & Phytosterol Data)
0.054	Cumin seed
0.054	Mustard seed, yellow
0.051	Cocoa Puffs, General Mills
0.049	Peppers, sweet, red, raw
0.043	Flaxseed
0.042	Zucchini, summer squash, w/ skin, boiled w/out salt, drained
0.042	Popcorn, regular butter flavor, microwave, made w/ partially hydrogenated oil (Missing Fats Data)
0.042	Mangos, raw
0.040	Chick peas (garbanzo, bengal gram), mature seeds, boiled, no salt
0.040	Egg, whole, cooked, scrambled
0.035	Raisins, seedless
0.035	Pinto beans, boiled, no salt, mature
0.034	Cream cheese (No Trans Fat Data)

0.034	Sausage, Italian, pork, cooked (No Trans Fat Data)
0.032	Cheerios, General Mills
0.031	White bread, commercially prepared (inlcudes soft crumbs)
0.030	Hummus, home prepared
0.030	Wheaties, General Mills
0.029	Eggplant, boiled, drained, no salt
0.028	Tomato sauce, canned
0.028	Potato, red, baked, flesh & skin
0.028	Cheddar cheese (No Trans Fat Data)
0.028	Ketchup
0.027	Walnuts, USDA A259, A257
0.027	Sunflower Seeds, hulled, dry roasted, no salt
0.027	Pretzels, soft
0.027	Wheat dinner rolls
0.027	American cheese, pasteurized, w/out disodium phosphate (No Trans Fat Data)
0.026	Peaches, raw
0.026	Papayas, raw
0.025	Cantaloupe, raw
0.025	Swiss Cheese (No Trans Fat Data)
0.024	FritoLay Sun Chips, Multi-grain snack, original flavor
0.024	Hot Sauce (ready-to-serve, sauce, pepper or hot)
0.024	Blue Cheese (No Trans Fat Data)
0.024	Avg. Cheese
0.023	Mozzarella cheese, whole milk (No Trans Fat Data)
0.023	Sweet potato, baked in skin, no salt
0.023	Kellogg's Raisin Bran
0.022	Avg. Seafood
0.022	Apple, raw, with skin A343
0.022	Provolone cheese (No Trans Fat Data)
0.022	Barley (hulled)
0.022	Strawberries, raw
0.021	Cherries, sweet, raw
0.021	Pretzels, hard, plain, salted
0.020	Potato, baked, flesh & skin, no salt
0.020	Potato, Russet, baked, flesh & skin

0.020	Puffed Wheat, Quaker
0.020	Mashed potatoes, home-prepared, whole milk & butter added
0.019	Whole wheat flour
0.019	Rice cakes, brown rice, plain
0.019	Parmesan cheese, grated (No Trans Fat Data)
0.019	Chocolate-flavored hazelnut spread (No Trans Fat Data)
0.019	Corn oil (vegetable oil), industrial and retail, all purpose salad or cooking
0.019	Candy bar, Snickers (King Size)
0.018	Avg. Cased Meat
0.018	Mustard, prepared, yellow
0.017	Lentils, mature seeds, boiled, no salt
0.017	Garlic, raw
0.016	Mozzarella cheese, part skim (No Trans Fat Data)
0.016	Hamburger patty, 80/20 ground chuck beef, broiled
0.016	Corned beef luncheon meat, beef, cured, canned (No Trans Fat Data)
0.014	Olives, pickled, canned or bottled, green
0.014	Whole wheat pita bread
0.014	Bran Flakes, single brand
0.013	Banana chips
0.013	Cheese-flavor puffs or twists, corn-based
0.013	Horseradish, prepared
0.013	Beef, eye of round, separable lean only, trimmed to 0" fat, all grades, roasted [cube steak]
0.013	Salami, cooked, beef (No Trans Fat Data)
0.013	Radishes, raw
0.012	Popcorn, air-popped
0.012	Lucky Charms, General Mills
0.012	Honey Smacks, Kellogg's
0.011	Popcorn, microwave, 94% fat free
0.011	Ricotta cheese, whole milk (No Trans Fat Data)
0.010	Butternut squash, winter, baked w/out salt, sugar or butter
0.010	Cranberry juice cocktail, bottled
0.009	Ice cream, soft-serve, french vanilla (No Trans Fat Data)
0.009	Ground turkey, cooked
0.009	Tilapia, cooked in dry heat

0.008	Spaghetti squash, winter, boiled w/out salt, drained
0.007	Pineapple, raw, all varieties
0.007	Pineapple, canned, juice pack, drained
0.007	Pastrami luncheon meat, beef, cured (No Trans Fat Data)
0.007	Peanut oil, salad or cooking (No Trans Fat or O3FA Data)
0.006	Brown rice, long-grain, cooked
0.006	Roll, hard, kaiser
0.005	Banana, raw
0.005	Coconut oil (Missing Trans Fat & O3FA Data)
0.005	Apple Jacks, Kellogg's
0.005	Peanut Butter Cap'n Crunch, Quaker
0.005	Cap'n Crunch with Crunch Berries, Quaker
0.005	Wild rice, cooked
0.005	Instant Oatmeal, Quaker, apples & cinnamon prepared w/ boiling water
0.004	Corn, sweet, yellow, boiled, drained, no salt
0.004	Avg. Lean Meat
0.004	Grape Juice, canned or bottled, unsweetened
0.004	Onion, raw
0.003	White flour, white, all-purpose, enriched, bleached
0.003	Matzo crackers, plain
0.003	Cap'n Crunch, Quaker
0.003	Ice creams, vanilla (No Trans Fat Data)
0.003	Bologna, lebanon, beef (No O3FA Data)
0.003	Oats, unenriched, boiled, w/out salt
0.003	Millet, cooked
0.003	Chicken, broilers or fryers, breast, meat only (no skin), roasted
0.002	Beets, raw
0.002	Milk, reduced fat, 2%, added Vit A
0.002	Milk, whole, 3.25% milkfat
0.002	Yogurt, regular low-fat, plain, 12 g protein per 8 oz
0.002	Beets, canned, drained solids
0.002	Coconut meat, raw
0.002	White pita bread, enriched
0.002	Frosted Flakes, Kellogg's
0.002	Scallops (bay & sea), steamed

0.002	Ginger, ground
0.001	Froot Loops, General Mills
0.001	Corn Pops, Kellogg's
0.001	Whiting, mixed species, cooked in dry heat
0.001	Bologna, chicken, pork, beef
0.001	Cocoa Krispies, Kellogg's (No O3FA Data)
0.001	Cottage cheese, 1% milkfat (No Trans Fat Data)
0.001	Cream of Wheat, instant, prepared with water and salt
0.001	Milk, lowfat, 1%, added Vit A
0.001	Oysters, eastern, wild, raw
0.001	Flounder (sole), cooked in dry heat
0.001	Coffee, brewed from grounds w/ tap water, no sugar or cream (No O3FA Data)
0.001	Lobster, northern, cooked in moist heat

Vitamin B1 (Thiamine)

Vitamin B1, mg/SS	Food
0.025	Wheaties, General Mills
0.021	Corn Flakes, Kellogg's
0.021	Frosted Flakes, Kellogg's
0.020	Cinnamon Toast Crunch cereal, ready-to-eat, General Mills
0.019	Cheerios, General Mills
0.018	Rice Krispies, Kellogg's
0.017	Lucky Charms, General Mills
0.017	Apple Jacks, Kellogg's
0.016	Flaxseed
0.016	Cap'n Crunch, Quaker
0.016	Cap'n Crunch with Crunch Berries, Quaker
0.015	Peanut Butter Cap'n Crunch, Quaker
0.015	Cocoa Krispies, Kellogg's (No O3FA Data)
0.014	Honey Smacks, Kellogg's
0.014	Golden Crisp, Post, Kraft
0.013	Bran Flakes, single brand
0.013	Cocoa Puffs, General Mills
0.013	Cilantro, dried (No O3FA Data)
0.013	Honeycomb cereal, Post, Kraft (low data)
0.012	Froot Loops, General Mills
0.012	Corn Pops, Kellogg's
0.012	Post Honey Bunches of Oats w/ Almonds (Missing Data)
0.011	Kellogg's Raisin Bran
0.010	Kellogg's Nutri-Grain Cereal Bars, fruit-filled
0.010	Kraft macaroni & cheese dinner, original, unprepared (Missing Data)
0.010	Salami, dry or hard, pork (No Trans Fat Data)
0.009	Pork tenderloin lean, roasted, URMIS 3358
0.009	Poppy seed
0.008	Pistachio nuts, dry roasted, no salt
0.008	White flour, white, all-purpose, enriched, bleached
0.008	Sage, ground
0.008	Oats
0.007	Macadamia nuts, dry roasted, with salt

0.007	Macadamia nuts, dry roasted, w/out salt
0.007	Barley (hulled)
0.006	Brazil nuts, dried, unblanched
0.006	White pita bread, enriched
0.006	Puffed Wheat, Quaker
0.006	Sausage, Italian, pork, cooked (No Trans Fat Data)
0.006	Ramen noodle soup, chicken flavor, dry
0.006	Cumin seed
0.006	Paprika
0.005	Pecans, dry roasted, no salt
0.005	White bread, commercially prepared (inlcudes soft crumbs)
0.005	Roll, hard, kaiser
0.005	Pretzels, hard, plain, salted
0.005	Bacon (pork), cured, cooked, pan-fried
0.005	Mustard seed, yellow
0.005	Thyme, dried
0.005	Rosemary, dried (Missing Data)
0.004	Avg. Nuts
0.004	Pretzels, soft
0.004	Whole wheat flour
0.004	Peanuts, dry roasted, no salt, all types
0.004	Soybeans (aka soy nuts) mature, dry roasted (Missing Sugar and Vitamin Data)
0.004	Wheat dinner rolls
0.004	Whole wheat bread, commecially prepared
0.004	Matzo crackers, plain
0.004	Ritz Crackers, Nabisco (Missing Vitamin Data)
0.004	Pepperoni, pork, beef
0.004	Caraway seed
0.004	Avg. Herbs
0.004	Dill weed, dried (Missing Data)
0.004	Fennel seed (Missing Vitamin & O3FA Data)
0.004	Pretzels, hard, whole-wheat (Missing Sugar Data)
0.004	Slice of pizza, fast food, pizza chain, 14", cheese topping, regular crust (No Trans Fat Data)
0.004	Mustard, prepared, yellow
0.003	Walnuts, USDA A259, A257

0.003	McDonald's French Fries
0.003	Egg noodles, cooked, enriched
0.003	Avg. Spice
0.003	Whole wheat bread, prepared from recipe
0.003	Whole wheat pita bread
0.003	Celery seed
0.003	Chili powder
0.003	Curry powder
0.003	Marjoram, dried
0.003	Oregano, dried
0.003	Anise seed (Missing Sugar, Vitamin, O3FA data)
0.003	Mace, ground (Missing Data)
0.003	Tarragon, dried (Missing Data)
0.003	Fenugreek seed (Missing Vitamin & O3, 6FA Data)
0.003	Nutmeg, ground (Missing O3FA Data)
0.003	Rye
0.003	Spaghetti, cooked, enriched w/out added salt, no sauce
0.003	Avg. Cased Meat
0.003	Peas, frozen, boiled, drained, no salt
0.003	Avg. Lean Meat
0.003	Salmon, Atlantic, wild, cooked in dry heat
0.003	Potato flour
0.002	Cream of Wheat, instant, prepared with water and salt
0.002	Corn, sweet, yellow, boiled, drained, no salt
0.002	Garlic, raw
0.002	Cashews, dry roasted, no salt
0.002	Almonds, USDA A256, A264
0.002	Instant Oatmeal, Quaker, apples & cinnamon prepared w/ boiling water
0.002	Cheese-flavor puffs or twists, corn-based
0.002	Granola bar, soft, uncoated, chocolate chip
0.002	Clams, mixed species, cooked in moist heat
0.002	Oysters, eastern, wild, cooked, moist heat
0.002	Turmeric, ground
0.002	Tortilla chips, plain, yellow corn (Missing Vitamin Data)
0.002	Cardamom (Missing Data)

0.002	Coriander seed (Missing Data)
0.002	Parsley, dried (Missing O3FA Data)
0.002	Cheetos Crunchy cheese-flavored snacks (No O3, 6FA Data)
0.002	Edamame beans, frozen, prepared
0.002	White rice, long-grain, regular, cooked
0.002	Parboiled rice, white, long-grain, enriched, cooked
0.002	Pinto beans, boiled, no salt, mature
0.002	Soybeans green, boiled, drained, no salt
0.002	Kidney beans, red, boiled, no salt, mature seeds
0.002	Bagel, plain, unenriched w/ calcium propionate, onion, poppy, sesame (no cream cheese)
0.002	Lentils, mature seeds, boiled, no salt
0.001	Asparagus, raw
0.001	Avg. Beans & Lentils
0.001	Turkey, stuffing, mashed potatoes w/ gravy, assorted vegetables, frozen, microwaved
0.001	Black beans, mature seeds, canned
0.001	Chick peas (garbanzo, bengal gram), mature seeds, boiled, no salt
0.001	Raisins, seedless
0.001	Milk chocolate candies (No Trans Fat Data)
0.001	Lima beans, immature, boiled, drained, no salt
0.001	Peanut butter, smooth, USDA Commodity
0.001	Millet, cooked
0.001	Orange, raw, all commercial varieties
0.001	Spinach, boiled, drained, no salt
0.001	Pineapple, canned, juice pack, drained
0.001	Quinoa, cooked
0.001	T-bone steak, short loin, beef trimmed to 1/8" fat, all grades, broiled
0.001	Brown rice, long-grain, cooked
0.001	Pomegranate, raw
0.001	Mushrooms, portabella, raw
0.001	Eggplant, boiled, drained, no salt
0.001	Cauliflower, raw
0.001	Romaine or cos lettuce
0.001	Cabbage, boiled, drained, no salt
0.001	Sweet potato, baked in skin, no salt

0.001	Banana chips
0.001	FritoLay Sun Chips, Multi-grain snack, original flavor
0.001	Pork-skins, plain
0.001	Sesame sticks, wheat-based, salted
0.001	Rice cakes, brown rice, plain
0.001	Popcorn, air-popped
0.001	Popcorn, microwave, 94% fat free
0.001	Popcorn, caramel-coated without peanuts
0.001	Margarine (vegetable oil spread, 70% fat, soybean & partially hydrogenated soybean, stick)
0.001	Egg, whole, cooked, scrambled
0.001	Beef, eye of round, separable lean only, trimmed to 0" fat, all grades, roasted [cube steak]
0.001	Ground turkey, cooked
0.001	Scallops (bay & sea), steamed
0.001	Tilapia, cooked in dry heat
0.001	Whiting, mixed species, cooked in dry heat
0.001	Anchovies, European, canned in oil, drained solids
0.001	Salami, cooked, beef (No Trans Fat Data)
0.001	Bologna, chicken, pork, beef
0.001	Pastrami luncheon meat, beef, cured (No Trans Fat Data)
0.001	Beef sticks, smoked (No Trans Fat Data)
0.001	Chocolate-flavored hazelnut spread (No Trans Fat Data)
0.001	Basil, dried
0.001	Cloves, ground
0.001	Black pepper
0.001	Spearmint, fresh (Missing Data)
0.001	Popcorn, regular butter flavor, microwave, made w/ partially hydrogenated oil (Missing Fats Data)
0.001	Bologna, lebanon, beef (No O3FA Data)
0.001	Allspice (Missing Data)
0.001	Saffron (Missing Data)
0.001	Salsa, USDA Commodity (Missing Sugar and Vitamin Data)
0.001	Mashed potatoes, home-prepared, whole milk & butter added
0.001	Candy bar, Snickers (King Size)
0.001	Oats, unenriched, boiled, w/out salt
0.001	Grits, corn, white, regular, quick, enriched, cooked with water,

	with salt
0.001	Avg. Leafy Green Vegetables
0.001	Hummus, home prepared
0.001	Oysters, eastern, wild, raw
0.001	Snap (green string) beans, boiled, drained, no salt
0.001	Flounder (sole), cooked in dry heat
0.001	Carrots, raw, USDA A099
0.001	Sunflower Seeds, hulled, dry roased, no salt
0.001	Kale, boiled, drained, no salt
0.001	Swiss Cheese (No Trans Fat Data)
0.001	Coconut meat, raw
0.001	Avg. Seafood
0.001	Broccoli, boiled, drained, no salt
0.001	Chicken, broilers or fryers, breast, meat only (no skin), roasted
0.001	Mushrooms, shiitake, cooked, no salt
0.001	Tomatoes, raw, red, ripe
0.001	Peppers, sweet, green, raw
0.001	Peppers, sweet, red, raw
0.001	Potato, baked, flesh & skin, no salt
0.001	Potato, red, baked, flesh & skin
0.001	Potato, Russet, baked, flesh & skin
0.001	Grapes, red or green, European type such as Thompson seedless, raw
0.001	Spaghetti squash, winter, boiled w/out salt, drained
0.001	Mushrooms, boiled, drained, no salt
0.001	Mushrooms, canned, drained solids
0.001	Avg. Vegetables
0.001	Onion, raw
0.001	Wild rice, cooked
0.001	Mangos, raw
0.001	Pineapple, raw, all varieties
0.001	Tuna fish, light, canned in water without salt, drained solids
0.001	White rice, long-grain, pre-cooked or instant, prepared (Missing O3FA Data)
0.001	Pak-choi, boiled, drained, no salt
0.001	Red snapper, cooked, dry heat
0.001	Swiss chard, boiled, drained, no salt

| 0.001 | Zucchini, summer squash, w/ skin, boiled w/out salt, drained |

Vitamin B2 (Riboflavin)

Vitamin B2, mg/SS	Food
0.028	Wheaties, General Mills
0.026	Corn Flakes, Kellogg's
0.023	Cocoa Krispies, Kellogg's (No O3FA Data)
0.022	Rice Krispies, Kellogg's
0.022	Apple Jacks, Kellogg's
0.020	Cinnamon Toast Crunch cereal, ready-to-eat, General Mills
0.019	Lucky Charms, General Mills
0.019	Frosted Flakes, Kellogg's
0.018	Cap'n Crunch, Quaker
0.018	Cap'n Crunch with Crunch Berries, Quaker
0.017	Peanut Butter Cap'n Crunch, Quaker
0.017	Paprika
0.016	Cheerios, General Mills
0.016	Kellogg's Raisin Bran
0.016	Honey Smacks, Kellogg's
0.016	Golden Crisp, Post, Kraft
0.015	Cilantro, dried (No O3FA Data)
0.015	Honeycomb cereal, Post, Kraft (low data)
0.014	Bran Flakes, single brand
0.014	Cocoa Puffs, General Mills
0.014	Corn Pops, Kellogg's
0.014	Post Honey Bunches of Oats w/ Almonds (Missing Data)
0.013	Froot Loops, General Mills
0.013	Tarragon, dried (Missing Data)
0.012	Parsley, dried (Missing O3FA Data)
0.011	Kellogg's Nutri-Grain Cereal Bars, fruit-filled
0.010	Almonds, USDA A256, A264
0.008	Chili powder
0.008	Soybeans (aka soy nuts) mature, dry roasted (Missing Sugar and Vitamin Data)
0.007	Corn chips, extruded, plain
0.006	Kraft macaroni & cheese dinner, original, unprepared (Missing Data)
0.005	Mushrooms, portabella, raw

0.005	Parmesan cheese, grated (No Trans Fat Data)
0.005	Thyme, fresh (Missing Data)
0.005	Slice of pizza, fast food, pizza chain, 14", cheese topping, regular crust (No Trans Fat Data)
0.005	White flour, white, all-purpose, enriched, bleached
0.005	Salmon, Atlantic, wild, cooked in dry heat
0.004	Avg. Spice
0.004	Puffed Wheat, Quaker
0.004	American cheese, pasteurized, w/out disodium phosphate (No Trans Fat Data)
0.004	Blue Cheese (No Trans Fat Data)
0.004	Egg, whole, cooked, scrambled
0.004	Pork tenderloin lean, roasted, URMIS 3358
0.004	Clams, mixed species, cooked in moist heat
0.004	Anchovies, European, canned in oil, drained solids
0.004	Beef sticks, smoked (No Trans Fat Data)
0.004	Caraway seed
0.004	Mustard seed, yellow
0.004	Thyme, dried
0.004	Velveeta cheese, Kraft, pasteurized spread (Missing Data)
0.004	Bay leaf (Missing Data)
0.004	Mace, ground (Missing Data)
0.004	Rosemary, dried (Missing Data)
0.004	Fennel seed (Missing Vitamin & O3FA Data)
0.004	Fenugreek seed (Missing Vitamin & O3, 6FA Data)
0.004	Cheddar cheese (No Trans Fat Data)
0.004	Salami, dry or hard, pork (No Trans Fat Data)
0.003	Mushrooms, boiled, drained, no salt
0.003	Avg. Cheese
0.003	Avg. Herbs
0.003	Swiss Cheese (No Trans Fat Data)
0.003	Provolone cheese (No Trans Fat Data)
0.003	White bread, commercially prepared (inlcudes soft crumbs)
0.003	Roll, hard, kaiser
0.003	Wheat dinner rolls
0.003	White pita bread, enriched
0.003	Matzo crackers, plain

0.003	Pretzels, hard, plain, salted
0.003	Pork-skins, plain
0.003	Ritz Crackers, Nabisco (Missing Vitamin Data)
0.003	Mozzarella cheese, part skim (No Trans Fat Data)
0.003	Bacon (pork), cured, cooked, pan-fried
0.003	Pepperoni, pork, beef
0.003	Ramen noodle soup, chicken flavor, dry
0.003	Basil, dried
0.003	Celery seed
0.003	Cloves, ground
0.003	Cumin seed
0.003	Curry powder
0.003	Marjoram, dried
0.003	Oregano, dried
0.003	Sage, ground
0.003	Anise seed (Missing Sugar, Vitamin, O3FA data)
0.003	Saffron (Missing Data)
0.003	Coriander seed (Missing Data)
0.003	Dill weed, dried (Missing Data)
0.003	Pretzels, hard, whole-wheat (Missing Sugar Data)
0.003	Milk chocolate candies (No Trans Fat Data)
0.003	Soybeans green, boiled, drained, no salt
0.003	Pretzels, soft
0.003	Barley (hulled)
0.003	Mozzarella cheese, whole milk (No Trans Fat Data)
0.003	Turkey, stuffing, mashed potatoes w/ gravy, assorted vegetables, frozen, microwaved
0.003	Whole wheat flour
0.002	Rye
0.002	Sunflower Seeds, hulled, dry roased, no salt
0.002	Avg. Nuts
0.002	Spinach, boiled, drained, no salt
0.002	Potato chips, plain, salted
0.002	Cashews, dry roasted, no salt
0.002	Avg. Lean Meat
0.002	T-bone steak, short loin, beef trimmed to 1/8" fat, all grades, broiled

0.002	Cream of Wheat, instant, prepared with water and salt
0.002	Milk, lowfat, 1%, added Vit A
0.002	Milk, reduced fat, 2%, added Vit A
0.002	Yogurt, regular low-fat, plain, 12 g protein per 8 oz
0.002	Instant Oatmeal, Quaker, apples & cinnamon prepared w/ boiling water
0.002	Flaxseed
0.002	Whole wheat bread, commecially prepared
0.002	Whole wheat bread, prepared from recipe
0.002	Cheese-flavor puffs or twists, corn-based
0.002	Rice cakes, brown rice, plain
0.002	Popcorn, microwave, 94% fat free
0.002	Ice creams, vanilla (No Trans Fat Data)
0.002	Ice cream, soft-serve, french vanilla (No Trans Fat Data)
0.002	Ricotta cheese, whole milk (No Trans Fat Data)
0.002	Beef, eye of round, separable lean only, trimmed to 0" fat, all grades, roasted [cube steak]
0.002	Hamburger patty, 80/20 ground chuck beef, broiled
0.002	Ground turkey, cooked
0.002	Oysters, eastern, wild, cooked, moist heat
0.002	Salami, cooked, beef (No Trans Fat Data)
0.002	Pastrami luncheon meat, beef, cured (No Trans Fat Data)
0.002	Sausage, Italian, pork, cooked (No Trans Fat Data)
0.002	Chocolate-flavored hazelnut spread (No Trans Fat Data)
0.002	Black pepper
0.002	Turmeric, ground
0.002	Rosemarry, fresh (Missing Data)
0.002	Spearmint, fresh (Missing Data)
0.002	Bologna, lebanon, beef (No O3FA Data)
0.002	Cardamom (Missing Data)
0.002	Cheetos Crunchy cheese-flavored snacks (No O3, 6FA Data)
0.002	Avg. Cased Meat
0.002	Cottage cheese, 1% milkfat (No Trans Fat Data)
0.002	Walnuts, USDA A259, A257
0.002	Milk, whole, 3.25% milkfat
0.002	Milk, nonfat, added Vit A
0.002	Pistachio nuts, dry roasted, no salt

0.002	Soy sauce (soy & wheat)
0.001	Avocado, raw, commercial varieties
0.001	Asparagus, raw
0.001	Avg. Seafood
0.001	Spaghetti, cooked, enriched w/out added salt, no sauce
0.001	Chicken, broilers or fryers, breast, meat only (no skin), roasted
0.001	Mushrooms, shiitake, cooked, no salt
0.001	Cream cheese (No Trans Fat Data)
0.001	Edamame beans, frozen, prepared
0.001	Oats
0.001	Black beans, mature seeds, canned
0.001	Egg noodles, cooked, enriched
0.001	Ketchup
0.001	Milk, nonfat, Ca fortified
0.001	Raisins, seedless
0.001	Peas, frozen, boiled, drained, no salt
0.001	Lima beans, immature, boiled, drained, no salt
0.001	Soy sauce, low sodium (soy & wheat)
0.001	Peanut butter, smooth, USDA Commodity
0.001	Swiss chard, boiled, drained, no salt
0.001	Quinoa, cooked
0.001	Broccoli, boiled, drained, no salt
0.001	Avg. Beans & Lentils
0.001	Pomegranate, raw
0.001	Cauliflower, raw
0.001	Romaine or cos lettuce
0.001	Sweet potato, baked in skin, no salt
0.001	Pecans, dry roasted, no salt
0.001	Whole wheat pita bread
0.001	Cake, snack cakes, crème-filled, chocolate with frosting
0.001	Tortilla chips, plain, white corn
0.001	Sesame sticks, wheat-based, salted
0.001	Popcorn, air-popped
0.001	Popcorn, caramel-coated without peanuts
0.001	Granola bar, soft, uncoated, chocolate chip
0.001	Hot Sauce (ready-to-serve, sauce, pepper or hot)

0.001	McDonald's spicy buffalo sauce
0.001	Turkey, fryer-roaster, breast meat only, roasted
0.001	Scallops (bay & sea), steamed
0.001	Crayfish, mixed species, farmed, cooked in moist heat
0.001	Tilapia, cooked in dry heat
0.001	Whiting, mixed species, cooked in dry heat
0.001	Bologna, chicken, pork, beef
0.001	Corned beef luncheon meat, beef, cured, canned (No Trans Fat Data)
0.001	Hotdog, Oscar Mayer Wiener, beef frank (No Trans Fat Data)
0.001	Ginger, ground
0.001	Poppy seed
0.001	Basil, fresh
0.001	Margarine, industrial, non-dairy, cottonseed, soy oil (partially hydrogenated), for flaky pastries
0.001	Popcorn, regular butter flavor, microwave, made w/ partially hydrogenated oil (Missing Fats Data)
0.001	Allspice (Missing Data)
0.001	Nutmeg, ground (Missing O3FA Data)
0.001	Pumpkin/Squash Seeds, dry roasted, no salt (Missing Vitamin & Se Data)
0.001	Acerola (West Indian cherry), raw (Missing Sugar and Vitamin Data)
0.001	Avg. Leafy Green Vegetables
0.001	Swordfish, cooked in dry heat
0.001	Dark chocolate candies, 60-69% cacao solids (Missing Vitamin Data)
0.001	Candy bar, Snickers (King Size)
0.001	Tomato sauce, canned
0.001	Oysters, eastern, wild, raw
0.001	Snap (green string) beans, boiled, drained, no salt
0.001	Flounder (sole), cooked in dry heat
0.001	Carrots, raw, USDA A099
0.001	Kale, boiled, drained, no salt
0.001	Bagel, plain, unenriched w/ calcium propionate, onion, poppy, sesame (no cream cheese)
0.001	Macadamia nuts, dry roasted, with salt
0.001	Macadamia nuts, dry roasted, w/out salt
0.001	Banana, raw

0.001	Garlic, raw
0.001	Beets, raw
0.001	Coffee, brewed from grounds w/ tap water, no sugar or cream (No O3FA Data)
0.001	Teriyaki sauce, ready-to-serve
0.001	Lobster, northern, cooked in moist heat
0.001	Peanuts, dry roasted, no salt, all types
0.001	Avg. Vegetables
0.001	Peppers, sweet, red, raw
0.001	Grapes, red or green, European type such as Thompson seedless, raw
0.001	Potato flour
0.001	Corn, sweet, yellow, boiled, drained, no salt
0.001	Chick peas (garbanzo, bengal gram), mature seeds, boiled, no salt
0.001	Wild rice, cooked
0.001	Mangos, raw
0.001	Pineapple, raw, all varieties
0.001	Tuna fish, light, canned in water without salt, drained solids
0.001	Pak-choi, boiled, drained, no salt
0.001	Pinto beans, boiled, no salt, mature
0.001	Tuna fish, white, canned in water without salt, drained solids
0.001	Millet, cooked
0.001	Peaches, raw
0.001	Kidney beans, red, boiled, no salt, mature seeds
0.001	Orange, raw, all commercial varieties
0.001	Zucchini, summer squash, w/ skin, boiled w/out salt, drained
0.001	Lentils, mature seeds, boiled, no salt

Vitamin B3 (Niacin)

Vitamin B3, mg/SS	Food
0.462	Barley (hulled)
0.333	Wheaties, General Mills
0.270	Apple Jacks, Kellogg's
0.268	Frosted Flakes, Kellogg's
0.244	Corn Flakes, Kellogg's
0.238	Cinnamon Toast Crunch cereal, ready-to-eat, General Mills
0.223	Lucky Charms, General Mills
0.213	Rice Krispies, Kellogg's
0.213	Cap'n Crunch, Quaker
0.213	Cap'n Crunch with Crunch Berries, Quaker
0.204	Peanut Butter Cap'n Crunch, Quaker
0.199	Anchovies, European, canned in oil, drained solids
0.191	Cheerios, General Mills
0.185	Honey Smacks, Kellogg's
0.185	Golden Crisp, Post, Kraft
0.172	Honeycomb cereal, Post, Kraft (low data)
0.167	Bran Flakes, single brand
0.167	Cocoa Puffs, General Mills
0.161	Corn Pops, Kellogg's
0.161	Post Honey Bunches of Oats w/ Almonds (Missing Data)
0.160	Cocoa Krispies, Kellogg's (No O3FA Data)
0.156	Froot Loops, General Mills
0.153	Paprika
0.147	Kellogg's Raisin Bran
0.137	Chicken, broilers or fryers, breast, meat only (no skin), roasted
0.135	Kellogg's Nutri-Grain Cereal Bars, fruit-filled
0.135	Peanuts, dry roasted, no salt, all types
0.133	Tuna fish, light, canned in water without salt, drained solids
0.132	Peanut butter, smooth, USDA Commodity
0.118	Swordfish, cooked in dry heat
0.116	Bacon (pork), cured, cooked, pan-fried
0.107	Cilantro, dried (No O3FA Data)
0.101	Salmon, Atlantic, wild, cooked in dry heat

0.090	Tarragon, dried (Missing Data)
0.085	Avg. Lean Meat
0.079	Chili powder
0.079	Mustard seed, yellow
0.079	Parsley, dried (Missing O3FA Data)
0.078	Rice cakes, brown rice, plain
0.075	Turkey, fryer-roaster, breast meat only, roasted
0.074	Pork tenderloin lean, roasted, URMIS 3358
0.070	Sunflower Seeds, hulled, dry roased, no salt
0.069	Basil, dried
0.065	Kraft macaroni & cheese dinner, original, unprepared (Missing Data)
0.065	Pretzels, hard, whole-wheat (Missing Sugar Data)
0.063	Whole wheat flour
0.062	Oregano, dried
0.061	Fennel seed (Missing Vitamin & O3FA Data)
0.060	Avg. Seafood
0.059	White flour, white, all-purpose, enriched, bleached
0.058	Tuna fish, white, canned in water without salt, drained solids
0.057	Sage, ground
0.056	Salami, dry or hard, pork (No Trans Fat Data)
0.056	Avg. Herbs
0.053	Puffed Wheat, Quaker
0.053	Beef, eye of round, separable lean only, trimmed to 0" fat, all grades, roasted [cube steak]
0.051	Pretzels, hard, plain, salted
0.051	Hamburger patty, 80/20 ground chuck beef, broiled
0.051	Turmeric, ground
0.050	Avg. Spice
0.049	Ritz Crackers, Nabisco (Missing Vitamin Data)
0.049	Thyme, dried
0.048	Ground turkey, cooked
0.047	Whole wheat bread, commecially prepared
0.047	Cheese-flavor puffs or twists, corn-based
0.047	Tilapia, cooked in dry heat
0.046	White pita bread, enriched
0.046	Pepperoni, pork, beef

0.046	Cumin seed
0.045	Mushrooms, portabella, raw
0.045	Beef sticks, smoked (No Trans Fat Data)
0.045	Mushrooms, boiled, drained, no salt
0.044	White bread, commercially prepared (inlcudes soft crumbs)
0.043	Pastrami luncheon meat, beef, cured (No Trans Fat Data)
0.043	Pretzels, soft
0.043	Rye
0.042	Roll, hard, kaiser
0.042	Sausage, Italian, pork, cooked (No Trans Fat Data)
0.042	Potato chips, plain, salted
0.041	T-bone steak, short loin, beef trimmed to 1/8" fat, all grades, broiled
0.041	Wheat dinner rolls
0.041	Marjoram, dried
0.040	Whole wheat bread, prepared from recipe
0.040	Ramen noodle soup, chicken flavor, dry
0.039	Matzo crackers, plain
0.038	Avg. Cased Meat
0.037	Avg. Nuts
0.036	Candy bar, Snickers (King Size)
0.036	Caraway seed
0.035	Bologna, chicken, pork, beef
0.035	Curry powder
0.035	Potato flour
0.034	Clams, mixed species, cooked in moist heat
0.034	Soy sauce, low sodium (soy & wheat)
0.034	Almonds, USDA A256, A264
0.033	Slice of pizza, fast food, pizza chain, 14", cheese topping, regular crust (No Trans Fat Data)
0.032	Salami, cooked, beef (No Trans Fat Data)
0.032	Bologna, lebanon, beef (No O3FA Data)
0.031	Cream of Wheat, instant, prepared with water and salt
0.031	Flaxseed
0.031	Celery seed
0.031	Anise seed (Missing Sugar, Vitamin, O3FA data)
0.031	Turkey, stuffing, mashed potatoes w/ gravy, assorted vegetables, frozen, microwaved

0.029	Allspice (Missing Data)
0.028	Whole wheat pita bread
0.028	Dill weed, dried (Missing Data)
0.028	Instant Oatmeal, Quaker, apples & cinnamon prepared w/ boiling water
0.027	McDonald's French Fries
0.026	Shrimp, mixed species, cooked in moist heat
0.025	Oysters, eastern, wild, cooked, moist heat
0.024	Corned beef luncheon meat, beef, cured, canned (No Trans Fat Data)
0.023	Popcorn, air-popped
0.023	Hotdog, Oscar Mayer Wiener, beef frank (No Trans Fat Data)
0.023	Cheetos Crunchy cheese-flavored snacks (No O3, 6FA Data)
0.023	Parboiled rice, white, long-grain, enriched, cooked
0.023	Macadamia nuts, dry roasted, with salt
0.023	Macadamia nuts, dry roasted, w/out salt
0.022	Flounder (sole), cooked in dry heat
0.022	Popcorn, caramel-coated without peanuts
0.022	Soy sauce (soy & wheat)
0.021	FritoLay Sun Chips, Multi-grain snack, original flavor
0.021	Popcorn, microwave, 94% fat free
0.021	Coriander seed (Missing Data)
0.021	Egg noodles, cooked, enriched
0.020	Bay leaf (Missing Data)
0.018	Thyme, fresh (Missing Data)
0.018	White rice, long-grain, pre-cooked or instant, prepared (Missing O3FA Data)
0.018	Bagel, plain, unenriched w/ calcium propionate, onion, poppy, sesame (no cream cheese)
0.017	Avocado, raw, commercial varieties
0.017	Spaghetti, cooked, enriched w/out added salt, no sauce
0.017	Crayfish, mixed species, farmed, cooked in moist heat
0.017	Whiting, mixed species, cooked in dry heat
0.017	Tortilla chips, plain, yellow corn (Missing Vitamin Data)
0.016	Potato, red, baked, flesh & skin
0.016	Mushrooms, canned, drained solids
0.016	Sesame sticks, wheat-based, salted
0.016	Popcorn, regular butter flavor, microwave, made w/ partially hydrogenated oil (Missing Fats Data)

0.016	Fenugreek seed (Missing Vitamin & O3, 6FA Data)
0.016	Corn, sweet, yellow, boiled, drained, no salt
0.015	Brown rice, long-grain, cooked
0.015	Mushrooms, shiitake, cooked, no salt
0.015	Sweet potato, baked in skin, no salt
0.015	Pork-skins, plain
0.015	Cloves, ground
0.015	Saffron (Missing Data)
0.015	Pistachio nuts, dry roasted, no salt
0.015	Peas, frozen, boiled, drained, no salt
0.015	White rice, long-grain, regular, cooked
0.014	Ketchup
0.014	Potato, baked, flesh & skin, no salt
0.014	Ginger, ground
0.014	Cashews, dry roasted, no salt
0.014	Oysters, eastern, wild, raw
0.013	Potato, Russet, baked, flesh & skin
0.013	Millet, cooked
0.013	Tortilla chips, plain, white corn
0.013	Scallops (bay & sea), steamed
0.013	Cinnamon
0.013	Mace, ground (Missing Data)
0.013	Nutmeg, ground (Missing O3FA Data)
0.013	Teriyaki sauce, ready-to-serve
0.013	Wild rice, cooked
0.012	Pecans, dry roasted, no salt
0.011	Walnuts, USDA A259, A257
0.011	Lobster, northern, cooked in moist heat
0.011	Black pepper
0.011	Cardamom (Missing Data)
0.011	Salsa, USDA Commodity (Missing Sugar and Vitamin Data)
0.011	Mashed potatoes, home-prepared, whole milk & butter added
0.011	Lentils, mature seeds, boiled, no salt
0.011	Lima beans, immature, boiled, drained, no salt
0.010	Soybeans (aka soy nuts) mature, dry roasted (Missing Sugar and Vitamin Data)

0.010	Carrots, raw, USDA A099
0.010	Peppers, sweet, red, raw
0.010	Blue Cheese (No Trans Fat Data)
0.010	Rosemary, dried (Missing Data)
0.010	Tomato sauce, canned
0.010	Butternut squash, winter, baked w/out salt, sugar or butter
0.010	Asparagus, raw
0.010	Oats
0.009	Edamame beans, frozen, prepared
0.009	Cake, snack cakes, crème-filled, chocolate with frosting
0.009	Poppy seed
0.009	Basil, fresh
0.009	Rosemarry, fresh (Missing Data)
0.009	Spearmint, fresh (Missing Data)
0.008	Spaghetti squash, winter, boiled w/out salt, drained
0.008	Milk, nonfat, added Vit A
0.008	Dark chocolate candies, 60-69% cacao solids (Missing Vitamin Data)
0.008	Peaches, raw
0.008	Granola bar, soft, uncoated, chocolate chip
0.008	Raisins, seedless
0.007	Garlic, raw
0.007	Grits, corn, white, regular, quick, enriched, cooked with water, with salt
0.007	Banana chips
0.007	McDonald's barbeque sauce
0.007	Avg. Beans & Lentils
0.007	Cantaloupe, raw
0.007	Banana, raw
0.006	Snap (green string) beans, boiled, drained, no salt
0.006	Avg. Vegetables
0.006	Black beans, mature seeds, canned
0.006	Mangos, raw
0.006	Tomatoes, raw, red, ripe
0.006	Eggplant, boiled, drained, no salt
0.006	Swanson chicken broth, 99% Fat Free
0.006	Raspberries, raw

0.006	Kidney beans, red, boiled, no salt, mature seeds
0.005	Chick peas (garbanzo, bengal gram), mature seeds, boiled, no salt
0.005	Broccoli, boiled, drained, no salt
0.005	Coconut meat, raw
0.005	Chicken noodle soup prepared with equal volume water
0.005	Mustard, prepared, yellow
0.005	Cauliflower, raw
0.005	Spinach, boiled, drained, no salt
0.005	Pineapple, raw, all varieties
0.005	Peppers, sweet, green, raw
0.005	Kale, boiled, drained, no salt
0.004	Zucchini, summer squash, w/ skin, boiled w/out salt, drained
0.004	Quinoa, cooked
0.004	Avg. Fruit
0.004	Pak-choi, boiled, drained, no salt
0.004	Soybeans green, boiled, drained, no salt
0.004	Hummus, home prepared
0.004	Blueberries, raw
0.004	Horseradish, prepared
0.004	McDonald's spicy buffalo sauce
0.004	Chocolate-flavored hazelnut spread (No Trans Fat Data)
0.004	Acerola (West Indian cherry), raw (Missing Sugar and Vitamin Data)
0.004	Strawberries, raw
0.004	Avg. Leafy Green Vegetables
0.004	Beets, raw
0.004	Papayas, raw
0.004	Milk chocolate candies (No Trans Fat Data)
0.004	Corn chips, extruded, plain
0.004	Red snapper, cooked, dry heat
0.003	Swiss chard, boiled, drained, no salt
0.003	Brazil nuts, dried, unblanched
0.003	Pomegranate, raw
0.003	Romaine or cos lettuce
0.003	Hot Sauce (ready-to-serve, sauce, pepper or hot)
0.003	Pumpkin/Squash Seeds, dry roasted, no salt (Missing Vitamin & Se Data)

0.003	Pinto beans, boiled, no salt, mature
0.003	White rice, glutinous, cooked
0.003	Orange, raw, all commercial varieties
0.003	Pineapple, canned, juice pack, drained
0.003	Radishes, raw
0.002	Oats, unenriched, boiled, w/out salt
0.002	Avg. Cheese
0.002	Cabbage, boiled, drained, no salt
0.002	Olives, pickled, canned or bottled, green
0.002	Grapes, red or green, European type such as Thompson seedless, raw
0.002	Coffee, brewed from grounds w/ tap water, no sugar or cream (No O3FA Data)
0.002	Beets, canned, drained solids
0.002	Provolone cheese (No Trans Fat Data)
0.001	Cherries, sweet, raw
0.001	Cottage cheese, 1% milkfat (No Trans Fat Data)
0.001	Cream cheese (No Trans Fat Data)
0.001	Pickles, cucumber, dill or kosher dill
0.001	Onion, raw
0.001	Chick peas (garbanzo, bengal gram), mature seeds, canned
0.001	Milk, whole, 3.25% milkfat
0.001	Yogurt, regular low-fat, plain, 12 g protein per 8 oz
0.001	Grape Juice, canned or bottled, unsweetened
0.001	Honey
0.001	Iceberg lettuce
0.001	Ice creams, vanilla (No Trans Fat Data)
0.001	Ice cream, soft-serve, french vanilla (No Trans Fat Data)
0.001	Ricotta cheese, whole milk (No Trans Fat Data)
0.001	American cheese, pasteurized, w/out disodium phosphate (No Trans Fat Data)
0.001	Parmesan cheese, grated (No Trans Fat Data)
0.001	Mozzarella cheese, part skim (No Trans Fat Data)
0.001	Egg, whole, cooked, scrambled
0.001	Margarine, industrial, non-dairy, cottonseed, soy oil (partially hydrogenated), for flaky pastries
0.001	Cucumber, raw w/ peel
0.001	Brown sugars

0.001	Apple, raw, with skin A343
0.001	Mozzarella cheese, whole milk (No Trans Fat Data)
0.001	Lemon juice, raw
0.001	Milk, lowfat, 1%, added Vit A
0.001	Milk, reduced fat, 2%, added Vit A
0.001	Milk, nonfat, Ca fortified
0.001	Apple Juice, canned or bottled, unsweetened
0.001	Cheddar cheese (No Trans Fat Data)
0.001	Swiss Cheese (No Trans Fat Data)
0.001	Rice noodles, cooked (Missing Sugar & Unsaturated Fat Data)

Vitamin B5 (Pantothenic Acid)

Vitamin B5, mg/SS	Food
0.070	Sunflower Seeds, hulled, dry roased, no salt
0.044	Potato chips, plain, salted
0.036	Mushrooms, shiitake, cooked, no salt
0.024	Lima beans, immature, boiled, drained, no salt
0.022	Mushrooms, boiled, drained, no salt
0.019	Salmon, Atlantic, wild, cooked in dry heat
0.018	Paprika
0.017	Blue Cheese (No Trans Fat Data)
0.015	Mushrooms, portabella, raw
0.015	Rye
0.015	Avg. Nuts
0.014	Avocado, raw, commercial varieties
0.014	Peanuts, dry roasted, no salt, all types
0.013	Oats
0.013	Bacon (pork), cured, cooked, pan-fried
0.012	Cashews, dry roasted, no salt
0.012	Tortilla chips, plain, white corn
0.012	Pepperoni, pork, beef
0.011	Cheerios, General Mills
0.011	Salami, dry or hard, pork (No Trans Fat Data)
0.010	Peanut butter, smooth, USDA Commodity
0.010	Flaxseed
0.010	Whole wheat flour
0.010	Cheese-flavor puffs or twists, corn-based
0.010	Rice cakes, brown rice, plain
0.010	Egg, whole, cooked, scrambled
0.010	Chicken, broilers or fryers, breast, meat only (no skin), roasted
0.010	Pork tenderloin lean, roasted, URMIS 3358
0.009	Sweet potato, baked in skin, no salt
0.009	FritoLay Sun Chips, Multi-grain snack, original flavor
0.009	Bran Flakes, single brand
0.009	Wheaties, General Mills
0.009	Kellogg's Raisin Bran

0.009	Anchovies, European, canned in oil, drained solids
0.009	Salami, cooked, beef (No Trans Fat Data)
0.009	Red snapper, cooked, dry heat
0.009	Corn, sweet, yellow, boiled, drained, no salt
0.008	Mushrooms, canned, drained solids
0.008	Avg. Lean Meat
0.008	Whole wheat pita bread
0.008	Ground turkey, cooked
0.008	Rosemarry, fresh (Missing Data)
0.008	Anise seed (Missing Sugar, Vitamin, O3FA data)
0.008	Pretzels, hard, whole-wheat (Missing Sugar Data)
0.007	Cauliflower, raw
0.007	Pecans, dry roasted, no salt
0.007	Whole wheat bread, commecially prepared
0.007	Lucky Charms, General Mills
0.007	Turkey, fryer-roaster, breast meat only, roasted
0.007	Hamburger patty, 80/20 ground chuck beef, broiled
0.007	Clams, mixed species, cooked in moist heat
0.007	Tilapia, cooked in dry heat
0.007	Bologna, chicken, pork, beef
0.007	McDonald's French Fries
0.007	Vegetable shortening, household, composite
0.007	Lentils, mature seeds, boiled, no salt
0.006	Avg. Cased Meat
0.006	Candy bar, Snickers (King Size)
0.006	Broccoli, boiled, drained, no salt
0.006	Macadamia nuts, dry roasted, with salt
0.006	Macadamia nuts, dry roasted, w/out salt
0.006	Banana chips
0.006	Rice Krispies, Kellogg's
0.006	Ice creams, vanilla (No Trans Fat Data)
0.006	Beef, eye of round, separable lean only, trimmed to 0" fat, all grades, roasted [cube steak]
0.006	Corned beef luncheon meat, beef, cured, canned (No Trans Fat Data)
0.006	Walnuts, USDA A259, A257
0.006	Garlic, raw

0.006	Avg. Seafood
0.006	Yogurt, regular low-fat, plain, 12 g protein per 8 oz
0.006	Cream cheese (No Trans Fat Data)
0.006	Corn chips, extruded, plain
0.006	Flounder (sole), cooked in dry heat
0.005	Avg. Cheese
0.005	Potato flour
0.005	Whole wheat bread, prepared from recipe
0.005	Popcorn, air-popped
0.005	Puffed Wheat, Quaker
0.005	Cinnamon Toast Crunch cereal, ready-to-eat, General Mills
0.005	Peanut Butter Cap'n Crunch, Quaker
0.005	Ice cream, soft-serve, french vanilla (No Trans Fat Data)
0.005	American cheese, pasteurized, w/out disodium phosphate (No Trans Fat Data)
0.005	Crayfish, mixed species, farmed, cooked in moist heat
0.005	Almonds, USDA A256, A264
0.005	Pistachio nuts, dry roasted, no salt
0.005	Milk chocolate candies (No Trans Fat Data)
0.005	Mashed potatoes, home-prepared, whole milk & butter added
0.005	Soybeans (aka soy nuts) mature, dry roasted (Missing Sugar and Vitamin Data)
0.005	Avg. Beans & Lentils
0.005	Swiss Cheese (No Trans Fat Data)
0.005	Provolone cheese (No Trans Fat Data)
0.004	Pomegranate, raw
0.004	White flour, white, all-purpose, enriched, bleached
0.004	Roll, hard, kaiser
0.004	Wheat dinner rolls
0.004	White pita bread, enriched
0.004	Matzo crackers, plain
0.004	Pork-skins, plain
0.004	Ritz Crackers, Nabisco (Missing Vitamin Data)
0.004	Honey Smacks, Kellogg's
0.004	Cap'n Crunch, Quaker
0.004	Cap'n Crunch with Crunch Berries, Quaker
0.004	Oysters, eastern, wild, cooked, moist heat

0.004	Chocolate-flavored hazelnut spread (No Trans Fat Data)
0.004	Cinnamon
0.004	Thyme, fresh (Missing Data)
0.004	Tortilla chips, plain, yellow corn (Missing Vitamin Data)
0.004	Slice of pizza, fast food, pizza chain, 14", cheese topping, regular crust (No Trans Fat Data)
0.004	Spaghetti squash, winter, boiled w/out salt, drained
0.004	Edamame beans, frozen, prepared
0.004	Bagel, plain, unenriched w/ calcium propionate, onion, poppy, sesame (no cream cheese)
0.004	White rice, long-grain, regular, cooked
0.004	Cheddar cheese (No Trans Fat Data)
0.004	Swordfish, cooked in dry heat
0.004	Milk, lowfat, 1%, added Vit A
0.004	Milk, reduced fat, 2%, added Vit A
0.004	Milk, whole, 3.25% milkfat
0.004	Potato, baked, flesh & skin, no salt
0.004	Potato, Russet, baked, flesh & skin
0.004	Banana, raw
0.004	Milk, nonfat, added Vit A
0.003	Butternut squash, winter, baked w/out salt, sugar or butter
0.003	Peppers, sweet, red, raw
0.003	Potato, red, baked, flesh & skin
0.003	Avg. Vegetables
0.003	Tomato sauce, canned
0.003	Raspberries, raw
0.003	Parboiled rice, white, long-grain, enriched, cooked
0.003	Soy sauce (soy & wheat)
0.003	Soy sauce, low sodium (soy & wheat)
0.003	T-bone steak, short loin, beef trimmed to 1/8" fat, all grades, broiled
0.003	Brown rice, long-grain, cooked
0.003	Chick peas (garbanzo, bengal gram), mature seeds, boiled, no salt
0.003	Coconut meat, raw
0.003	Pretzels, hard, plain, salted
0.003	Granola bar, soft, uncoated, chocolate chip
0.003	Froot Loops, General Mills

0.003	Apple Jacks, Kellogg's
0.003	Corn Pops, Kellogg's
0.003	Parmesan cheese, grated (No Trans Fat Data)
0.003	Shrimp, mixed species, cooked in moist heat
0.003	Whiting, mixed species, cooked in dry heat
0.003	Pastrami luncheon meat, beef, cured (No Trans Fat Data)
0.003	Beef sticks, smoked (No Trans Fat Data)
0.003	Poppy seed
0.003	Spearmint, fresh (Missing Data)
0.003	Popcorn, regular butter flavor, microwave, made w/ partially hydrogenated oil (Missing Fats Data)
0.003	Bologna, lebanon, beef (No O3FA Data)
0.003	Acerola (West Indian cherry), raw (Missing Sugar and Vitamin Data)
0.003	Oats, unenriched, boiled, w/out salt
0.003	Asparagus, raw
0.003	Chick peas (garbanzo, bengal gram), mature seeds, canned
0.003	Hummus, home prepared
0.003	Mustard, prepared, yellow
0.003	Orange, raw, all commercial varieties
0.003	Lobster, northern, cooked in moist heat
0.003	Barley (hulled)
0.003	Dark chocolate candies, 60-69% cacao solids (Missing Vitamin Data)
0.003	Cucumber, raw w/ peel
0.003	Egg noodles, cooked, enriched
0.002	Pineapple, raw, all varieties
0.002	Tuna fish, light, canned in water without salt, drained solids
0.002	Carrots, raw, USDA A099
0.002	Pinto beans, boiled, no salt, mature
0.002	Turkey, stuffing, mashed potatoes w/ gravy, assorted vegetables, frozen, microwaved
0.002	White rice, glutinous, cooked
0.002	Kidney beans, red, boiled, no salt, mature seeds
0.002	Cottage cheese, 1% milkfat (No Trans Fat Data)
0.002	Coffee, brewed from grounds w/ tap water, no sugar or cream (No O3FA Data)
0.002	Cherries, sweet, raw

0.002	Papayas, raw
0.002	Teriyaki sauce, ready-to-serve
0.002	Avg. Fruit
0.002	Oysters, eastern, wild, raw
0.002	Cabbage, boiled, drained, no salt
0.002	White bread, commercially prepared (inlcudes soft crumbs)
0.002	Sesame sticks, wheat-based, salted
0.002	McDonald's barbeque sauce
0.002	Cocoa Puffs, General Mills
0.002	Frosted Flakes, Kellogg's
0.002	Ricotta cheese, whole milk (No Trans Fat Data)
0.002	Hotdog, Oscar Mayer Wiener, beef frank (No Trans Fat Data)
0.002	Ramen noodle soup, chicken flavor, dry
0.002	Basil, fresh
0.002	Avg. Spice
0.002	Margarine, industrial, non-dairy, cottonseed, soy oil (partially hydrogenated), for flaky pastries
0.002	Cocoa Krispies, Kellogg's (No O3FA Data)
0.002	Avg. Leafy Green Vegetables
0.002	Wild rice, cooked
0.002	Mangos, raw
0.002	Mayonnaise, soybean oil, w/ salt (salad dressing)
0.002	Mozzarella cheese, whole milk (No Trans Fat Data)
0.002	Soybeans green, boiled, drained, no salt
0.002	Radishes, raw
0.002	Millet, cooked
0.002	Peaches, raw
0.002	Swiss chard, boiled, drained, no salt
0.002	Beets, canned, drained solids
0.002	Black beans, mature seeds, canned
0.002	Spinach, boiled, drained, no salt
0.002	Peas, frozen, boiled, drained, no salt
0.002	Brazil nuts, dried, unblanched
0.001	Beets, raw
0.001	Spaghetti, cooked, enriched w/out added salt, no sauce
0.001	Brown sugars

0.001	Instant Oatmeal, Quaker, apples & cinnamon prepared w/ boiling water
0.001	Swanson chicken broth, 99% Fat Free
0.001	Strawberries, raw
0.001	Onion, raw
0.001	Lemon juice, raw
0.001	Raisins, seedless
0.001	Tuna fish, white, canned in water without salt, drained solids
0.001	Zucchini, summer squash, w/ skin, boiled w/out salt, drained
0.001	Blueberries, raw
0.001	Eggplant, boiled, drained, no salt
0.001	Iceberg lettuce
0.001	Romaine or cos lettuce
0.001	Cake, snack cakes, crème-filled, chocolate with frosting
0.001	Popcorn, caramel-coated without peanuts
0.001	Hot Sauce (ready-to-serve, sauce, pepper or hot)
0.001	Horseradish, prepared
0.001	Light mayo (salad dressing)
0.001	McDonald's spicy buffalo sauce
0.001	Corn Flakes, Kellogg's
0.001	Mozzarella cheese, part skim (No Trans Fat Data)
0.001	Pumpkin/Squash Seeds, dry roasted, no salt (Missing Vitamin & Se Data)
0.001	Cantaloupe, raw
0.001	Butter, salted (No Trans Fat Data)
0.001	Cream of Wheat, instant, prepared with water and salt
0.001	Grits, corn, white, regular, quick, enriched, cooked with water, with salt
0.001	Chicken noodle soup prepared with equal volume water
0.001	Snap (green string) beans, boiled, drained, no salt
0.001	Kale, boiled, drained, no salt
0.001	Tomatoes, raw, red, ripe
0.001	Peppers, sweet, green, raw
0.001	Grapes, red or green, European type such as Thompson seedless, raw
0.001	Pickles, cucumber, dill or kosher dill
0.001	White rice, long-grain, pre-cooked or instant, prepared (Missing O3FA Data)

0.001	Honey
0.001	Pak-choi, boiled, drained, no salt

Vitamin B6 (Pyridoxine)

Vitamin B6, mg/SS	Food
0.040	Paprika
0.037	Chili powder
0.034	Corn Flakes, Kellogg's
0.033	Wheaties, General Mills
0.033	Cocoa Krispies, Kellogg's (No O3FA Data)
0.030	Rice noodles, cooked (Missing Sugar & Unsaturated Fat Data)
0.030	Rice Krispies, Kellogg's
0.029	Frosted Flakes, Kellogg's
0.027	Sage, ground
0.025	Apple Jacks, Kellogg's
0.024	Tarragon, dried (Missing Data)
0.023	Basil, dried
0.021	Cap'n Crunch, Quaker
0.021	Cap'n Crunch with Crunch Berries, Quaker
0.020	Peanut Butter Cap'n Crunch, Quaker
0.019	Lucky Charms, General Mills
0.019	Honey Smacks, Kellogg's
0.019	Golden Crisp, Post, Kraft
0.018	Cheerios, General Mills
0.018	Kellogg's Raisin Bran
0.018	Cinnamon Toast Crunch cereal, ready-to-eat, General Mills
0.018	Turmeric, ground
0.017	Bran Flakes, single brand
0.017	Cocoa Puffs, General Mills
0.017	Bay leaf (Missing Data)
0.017	Rosemary, dried (Missing Data)
0.017	Dill weed, dried (Missing Data)
0.017	Honeycomb cereal, Post, Kraft (low data)
0.016	Froot Loops, General Mills
0.016	Corn Pops, Kellogg's
0.016	Post Honey Bunches of Oats w/ Almonds (Missing Data)
0.016	Avg. Herbs
0.014	Kellogg's Nutri-Grain Cereal Bars, fruit-filled

0.013	Pistachio nuts, dry roasted, no salt
0.013	Avg. Spice
0.013	Garlic, raw
0.012	Curry powder
0.012	Marjoram, dried
0.012	Oregano, dried
0.010	Saffron (Missing Data)
0.010	Parsley, dried (Missing O3FA Data)
0.010	Salmon, Atlantic, wild, cooked in dry heat
0.009	Celery seed
0.008	Sunflower Seeds, hulled, dry roasted, no salt
0.008	Potato flour
0.007	Potato chips, plain, salted
0.007	Pork tenderloin lean, roasted, URMIS 3358
0.007	Anise seed (Missing Sugar, Vitamin, O3FA data)
0.006	Turkey, fryer-roaster, breast meat only, roasted
0.006	Cloves, ground
0.006	Cilantro, dried (No O3FA Data)
0.006	Fenugreek seed (Missing Vitamin & O3, 6FA Data)
0.006	Mayonnaise, soybean oil, w/ salt (salad dressing)
0.006	Chicken, broilers or fryers, breast, meat only (no skin), roasted
0.006	Avg. Lean Meat
0.005	Peanut butter, smooth, USDA Commodity
0.005	Salami, dry or hard, pork (No Trans Fat Data)
0.005	Walnuts, USDA A259, A257
0.005	McDonald's French Fries
0.005	Flaxseed
0.005	Thyme, dried
0.005	Fennel seed (Missing Vitamin & O3FA Data)
0.005	Avg. Nuts
0.005	Red snapper, cooked, dry heat
0.005	Chick peas (garbanzo, bengal gram), mature seeds, canned
0.004	Hummus, home prepared
0.004	Beef, eye of round, separable lean only, trimmed to 0" fat, all grades, roasted [cube steak]
0.004	Hamburger patty, 80/20 ground chuck beef, broiled

0.004	Ground turkey, cooked
0.004	Bacon (pork), cured, cooked, pan-fried
0.004	Pepperoni, pork, beef
0.004	Caraway seed
0.004	Cumin seed
0.004	Mustard seed, yellow
0.004	Bologna, lebanon, beef (No O3FA Data)
0.004	Macadamia nuts, dry roasted, with salt
0.004	Macadamia nuts, dry roasted, w/out salt
0.004	Swordfish, cooked in dry heat
0.004	Potato, Russet, baked, flesh & skin
0.004	Banana, raw
0.004	Tuna fish, light, canned in water without salt, drained solids
0.003	T-bone steak, short loin, beef trimmed to 1/8" fat, all grades, broiled
0.003	Whole wheat flour
0.003	Barley (hulled)
0.003	Potato, baked, flesh & skin, no salt
0.003	Sweet potato, baked in skin, no salt
0.003	Whole wheat pita bread
0.003	Banana chips
0.003	Sausage, Italian, pork, cooked (No Trans Fat Data)
0.003	Black pepper
0.003	Rosemarry, fresh (Missing Data)
0.003	Thyme, fresh (Missing Data)
0.003	Pretzels, hard, whole-wheat (Missing Sugar Data)
0.003	Rye
0.003	Cashews, dry roasted, no salt
0.003	Cream of Wheat, instant, prepared with water and salt
0.003	Peanuts, dry roasted, no salt, all types
0.003	Peppers, sweet, red, raw
0.003	Instant Oatmeal, Quaker, apples & cinnamon prepared w/ boiling water
0.003	Avg. Seafood
0.003	Avg. Cased Meat
0.002	Avocado, raw, commercial varieties
0.002	Mashed potatoes, home-prepared, whole milk & butter added

0.002	Flounder (sole), cooked in dry heat
0.002	Pinto beans, boiled, no salt, mature
0.002	Soybeans green, boiled, drained, no salt
0.002	Tuna fish, white, canned in water without salt, drained solids
0.002	Soybeans (aka soy nuts) mature, dry roasted (Missing Sugar and Vitamin Data)
0.002	Spinach, boiled, drained, no salt
0.002	Broccoli, boiled, drained, no salt
0.002	Lentils, mature seeds, boiled, no salt
0.002	Peppers, sweet, green, raw
0.002	Potato, red, baked, flesh & skin
0.002	Cauliflower, raw
0.002	Pecans, dry roasted, no salt
0.002	Whole wheat bread, commecially prepared
0.002	Whole wheat bread, prepared from recipe
0.002	Tortilla chips, plain, white corn
0.002	FritoLay Sun Chips, Multi-grain snack, original flavor
0.002	Rice cakes, brown rice, plain
0.002	Popcorn, air-popped
0.002	Popcorn, microwave, 94% fat free
0.002	Hot Sauce (ready-to-serve, sauce, pepper or hot)
0.002	McDonald's spicy buffalo sauce
0.002	Blue Cheese (No Trans Fat Data)
0.002	Whiting, mixed species, cooked in dry heat
0.002	Anchovies, European, canned in oil, drained solids
0.002	Salami, cooked, beef (No Trans Fat Data)
0.002	Bologna, chicken, pork, beef
0.002	Pastrami luncheon meat, beef, cured (No Trans Fat Data)
0.002	Beef sticks, smoked (No Trans Fat Data)
0.002	Cinnamon
0.002	Ginger, ground
0.002	Poppy seed
0.002	Basil, fresh
0.002	Spearmint, fresh (Missing Data)
0.002	Popcorn, regular butter flavor, microwave, made w/ partially hydrogenated oil (Missing Fats Data)

0.002	Tortilla chips, plain, yellow corn (Missing Vitamin Data)
0.002	Allspice (Missing Data)
0.002	Cardamom (Missing Data)
0.002	Mace, ground (Missing Data)
0.002	Nutmeg, ground (Missing O3FA Data)
0.002	Raisins, seedless
0.002	Turkey, stuffing, mashed potatoes w/ gravy, assorted vegetables, frozen, microwaved
0.002	Pak-choi, boiled, drained, no salt
0.002	Lima beans, immature, boiled, drained, no salt
0.002	Avg. Beans & Lentils
0.002	Ketchup
0.002	Soy sauce (soy & wheat)
0.002	Soy sauce, low sodium (soy & wheat)
0.002	Carrots, raw, USDA A099
0.002	Kale, boiled, drained, no salt
0.002	Brown rice, long-grain, cooked
0.001	Avg. Vegetables
0.001	Butternut squash, winter, baked w/out salt, sugar or butter
0.001	Avg. Leafy Green Vegetables
0.001	Almonds, USDA A256, A264
0.001	Mushrooms, shiitake, cooked, no salt
0.001	Spaghetti squash, winter, boiled w/out salt, drained
0.001	Edamame beans, frozen, prepared
0.001	Oats
0.001	Parboiled rice, white, long-grain, enriched, cooked
0.001	Onion, raw
0.001	Chick peas (garbanzo, bengal gram), mature seeds, boiled, no salt
0.001	Wild rice, cooked
0.001	Mangos, raw
0.001	Pineapple, raw, all varieties
0.001	Peas, frozen, boiled, drained, no salt
0.001	Millet, cooked
0.001	Kidney beans, red, boiled, no salt, mature seeds
0.001	Quinoa, cooked
0.001	Teriyaki sauce, ready-to-serve

0.001	Corn chips, extruded, plain
0.001	Pomegranate, raw
0.001	Blueberries, raw
0.001	Mushrooms, portabella, raw
0.001	Eggplant, boiled, drained, no salt
0.001	Romaine or cos lettuce
0.001	Cabbage, boiled, drained, no salt
0.001	White bread, commercially prepared (inlcudes soft crumbs)
0.001	Wheat dinner rolls
0.001	Matzo crackers, plain
0.001	Cake, snack cakes, crème-filled, chocolate with frosting
0.001	Cheese-flavor puffs or twists, corn-based
0.001	Sesame sticks, wheat-based, salted
0.001	Ritz Crackers, Nabisco (Missing Vitamin Data)
0.001	Granola bar, soft, uncoated, chocolate chip
0.001	Horseradish, prepared
0.001	McDonald's barbeque sauce
0.001	Puffed Wheat, Quaker
0.001	American cheese, pasteurized, w/out disodium phosphate (No Trans Fat Data)
0.001	Mozzarella cheese, part skim (No Trans Fat Data)
0.001	Egg, whole, cooked, scrambled
0.001	Shrimp, mixed species, cooked in moist heat
0.001	Scallops (bay & sea), steamed
0.001	Clams, mixed species, cooked in moist heat
0.001	Oysters, eastern, wild, cooked, moist heat
0.001	Crayfish, mixed species, farmed, cooked in moist heat
0.001	Tilapia, cooked in dry heat
0.001	Corned beef luncheon meat, beef, cured, canned (No Trans Fat Data)
0.001	Hotdog, Oscar Mayer Wiener, beef frank (No Trans Fat Data)
0.001	Chocolate-flavored hazelnut spread (No Trans Fat Data)
0.001	Ramen noodle soup, chicken flavor, dry
0.001	Salsa, USDA Commodity (Missing Sugar and Vitamin Data)
0.001	Cantaloupe, raw
0.001	Slice of pizza, fast food, pizza chain, 14", cheese topping, regular crust (No Trans Fat Data)

0.001	Avg. Fruit
0.001	Candy bar, Snickers (King Size)
0.001	Cottage cheese, 1% milkfat (No Trans Fat Data)
0.001	Radishes, raw
0.001	Tomato sauce, canned
0.001	Raspberries, raw
0.001	Oysters, eastern, wild, raw
0.001	Mustard, prepared, yellow
0.001	Snap (green string) beans, boiled, drained, no salt
0.001	White flour, white, all-purpose, enriched, bleached
0.001	Bagel, plain, unenriched w/ calcium propionate, onion, poppy, sesame (no cream cheese)
0.001	Cheddar cheese (No Trans Fat Data)
0.001	Swiss Cheese (No Trans Fat Data)
0.001	Provolone cheese (No Trans Fat Data)
0.001	Brazil nuts, dried, unblanched
0.001	Asparagus, raw
0.001	Beets, raw
0.001	Cherries, sweet, raw
0.001	Spaghetti, cooked, enriched w/out added salt, no sauce
0.001	Lobster, northern, cooked in moist heat
0.001	Beets, canned, drained solids
0.001	Tomatoes, raw, red, ripe
0.001	Grapes, red or green, European type such as Thompson seedless, raw
0.001	Strawberries, raw
0.001	Mushrooms, boiled, drained, no salt
0.001	Mushrooms, canned, drained solids
0.001	Avg. Cheese
0.001	White rice, long-grain, regular, cooked
0.001	Egg noodles, cooked, enriched
0.001	Corn, sweet, yellow, boiled, drained, no salt
0.001	White rice, long-grain, pre-cooked or instant, prepared (Missing O3FA Data)
0.001	Milk chocolate candies (No Trans Fat Data)
0.001	Swiss chard, boiled, drained, no salt
0.001	Orange, raw, all commercial varieties
0.001	Zucchini, summer squash, w/ skin, boiled w/out salt, drained

0.001	Pineapple, canned, juice pack, drained
0.001	Coconut meat, raw

Vitamin B9 (Folate or Folic Acid)

Vitamin B9, ug/SS	Food
15.550	Cap'n Crunch, Quaker
15.540	Peanut Butter Cap'n Crunch, Quaker
15.390	Cap'n Crunch with Crunch Berries, Quaker
9.750	Cheerios, General Mills
7.450	Lucky Charms, General Mills
6.670	Wheaties, General Mills
6.370	Cocoa Krispies, Kellogg's (No O3FA Data)
5.390	Rice Krispies, Kellogg's
4.800	Corn Flakes, Kellogg's
3.960	Apple Jacks, Kellogg's
3.820	Frosted Flakes, Kellogg's
3.760	Cinnamon Toast Crunch cereal, ready-to-eat, General Mills
3.750	Honey Smacks, Kellogg's
3.700	Golden Crisp, Post, Kraft
3.450	Honeycomb cereal, Post, Kraft (low data)
3.330	Bran Flakes, single brand
3.330	Cocoa Puffs, General Mills
3.290	Corn Pops, Kellogg's
3.230	Post Honey Bunches of Oats w/ Almonds (Missing Data)
3.130	Froot Loops, General Mills
3.110	Edamame beans, frozen, prepared
3.070	Rosemary, dried (Missing Data)
2.740	Basil, dried
2.740	Marjoram, dried
2.740	Oregano, dried
2.740	Sage, ground
2.740	Thyme, dried
2.740	Avg. Herbs
2.740	Tarragon, dried (Missing Data)
2.740	Cilantro, dried (No O3FA Data)
2.550	Kellogg's Raisin Bran
2.367	Sunflower Seeds, hulled, dry roasted, no salt
2.052	Soybeans (aka soy nuts) mature, dry roasted (Missing Sugar and

	Vitamin Data)
1.860	Pretzels, hard, plain, salted
1.832	White flour, white, all-purpose, enriched, bleached
1.808	Lentils, mature seeds, boiled, no salt
1.800	Bay leaf (Missing Data)
1.800	Parsley, dried (Missing O3FA Data)
1.720	Chick peas (garbanzo, bengal gram), mature seeds, boiled, no salt
1.719	Pinto beans, boiled, no salt, mature
1.540	Puffed Wheat, Quaker
1.540	Curry powder
1.461	Spinach, boiled, drained, no salt
1.452	Peanuts, dry roasted, no salt, all types
1.360	Romaine or cos lettuce
1.299	Kidney beans, red, boiled, no salt, mature seeds
1.170	Ramen noodle soup, chicken flavor, dry
1.150	Avg. Beans & Lentils
1.110	White bread, commercially prepared (inlcudes soft crumbs)
1.090	Rosemarry, fresh (Missing Data)
1.088	Beets, raw
1.080	Kellogg's Nutri-Grain Cereal Bars, fruit-filled
1.079	Broccoli, boiled, drained, no salt
1.070	White pita bread, enriched
1.060	Paprika
1.050	Spearmint, fresh (Missing Data)
1.000	Chili powder
0.983	Walnuts, USDA A259, A257
0.950	Roll, hard, kaiser
0.930	Slice of pizza, fast food, pizza chain, 14", cheese topping, regular crust (No Trans Fat Data)
0.930	Cloves, ground
0.930	Kraft macaroni & cheese dinner, original, unprepared (Missing Data)
0.930	Saffron (Missing Data)
0.870	Flaxseed
0.838	Egg noodles, cooked, enriched
0.820	Poppy seed
0.811	Avocado, raw, commercial varieties

0.810	Parboiled rice, white, long-grain, enriched, cooked
0.761	Avg. Nuts
0.760	Mustard seed, yellow
0.760	Mace, ground (Missing Data)
0.760	Nutmeg, ground (Missing O3FA Data)
0.749	Potato chips, plain, salted
0.729	Spaghetti, cooked, enriched w/out added salt, no sauce
0.720	Ritz Crackers, Nabisco (Missing Vitamin Data)
0.697	White rice, long-grain, pre-cooked or instant, prepared (Missing O3FA Data)
0.690	Avg. Leafy Green Vegetables
0.690	Cashews, dry roasted, no salt
0.680	Basil, fresh
0.671	Chick peas (garbanzo, bengal gram), mature seeds, canned
0.650	Whole wheat bread, prepared from recipe
0.618	Cream of Wheat, instant, prepared with water and salt
0.608	Black beans, mature seeds, canned
0.600	Wheat dinner rolls
0.600	McDonald's French Fries
0.598	Rye
0.589	Hummus, home prepared
0.589	Peas, frozen, boiled, drained, no salt
0.580	White rice, long-grain, regular, cooked
0.570	Cauliflower, raw
0.570	Horseradish, prepared
0.570	Fenugreek seed (Missing Vitamin & O3, 6FA Data)
0.570	Instant Oatmeal, Quaker, apples & cinnamon prepared w/ boiling water
0.560	Oats
0.558	Avg. Spice
0.550	Cheese-flavor puffs or twists, corn-based
0.540	Soybeans green, boiled, drained, no salt
0.540	Pretzels, hard, whole-wheat (Missing Sugar Data)
0.520	Asparagus, raw
0.500	Almonds, USDA A256, A264
0.500	Pistachio nuts, dry roasted, no salt
0.500	Whole wheat bread, commecially prepared

0.460	Corn, sweet, yellow, boiled, drained, no salt
0.460	Peppers, sweet, red, raw
0.450	Thyme, fresh (Missing Data)
0.440	Whole wheat flour
0.420	Quinoa, cooked
0.410	Pak-choi, boiled, drained, no salt
0.391	Avg. Vegetables
0.390	Turmeric, ground
0.380	Pomegranate, raw
0.380	Papayas, raw
0.360	Blue Cheese (No Trans Fat Data)
0.360	Allspice (Missing Data)
0.350	Whole wheat pita bread
0.350	Peanut butter, smooth, USDA Commodity
0.330	Snap (green string) beans, boiled, drained, no salt
0.310	Popcorn, air-popped
0.307	Orange, raw, all commercial varieties
0.300	Cabbage, boiled, drained, no salt
0.300	Egg, whole, cooked, scrambled
0.300	Beets, canned, drained solids
0.290	Salmon, Atlantic, wild, cooked in dry heat
0.290	Iceberg lettuce
0.290	Clams, mixed species, cooked in moist heat
0.280	Potato, baked, flesh & skin, no salt
0.270	Candy bar, Snickers (King Size)
0.270	Potato, red, baked, flesh & skin
0.260	Lima beans, immature, boiled, drained, no salt
0.260	Cake, snack cakes, crème-filled, chocolate with frosting
0.260	Potato, Russet, baked, flesh & skin
0.260	Wild rice, cooked
0.259	Coconut meat, raw
0.250	Radishes, raw
0.250	Potato flour
0.250	FritoLay Sun Chips, Multi-grain snack, original flavor
0.240	Strawberries, raw
0.240	Turkey, stuffing, mashed potatoes w/ gravy, assorted vegetables,

	frozen, microwaved
0.240	Pretzels, soft
0.220	Brazil nuts, dried, unblanched
0.220	Mushrooms, portabella, raw
0.220	Sesame sticks, wheat-based, salted
0.220	Bagel, plain, unenriched w/ calcium propionate, onion, poppy, sesame (no cream cheese)
0.210	Mushrooms, shiitake, cooked, no salt
0.210	Rice cakes, brown rice, plain
0.210	Cantaloupe, raw
0.210	Raspberries, raw
0.200	Tortilla chips, plain, white corn
0.200	Banana, raw
0.190	Millet, cooked
0.190	Barley (hulled)
0.190	Onion, raw
0.190	Salsa, USDA Commodity (Missing Sugar and Vitamin Data)
0.190	Carrots, raw, USDA A099
0.190	Butternut squash, winter, baked w/out salt, sugar or butter
0.180	Cheddar cheese (No Trans Fat Data)
0.180	Mushrooms, boiled, drained, no salt
0.180	Pineapple, raw, all varieties
0.180	Popcorn, microwave, 94% fat free
0.174	Avg. Fruit
0.170	Zucchini, summer squash, w/ skin, boiled w/out salt, drained
0.170	Matzo crackers, plain
0.160	Pecans, dry roasted, no salt
0.160	Granola bar, soft, uncoated, chocolate chip
0.160	Soy sauce, low sodium (soy & wheat)
0.150	Whiting, mixed species, cooked in dry heat
0.150	Popcorn, regular butter flavor, microwave, made w/ partially hydrogenated oil (Missing Fats Data)
0.150	Tomatoes, raw, red, ripe
0.140	Mangos, raw
0.140	Eggplant, boiled, drained, no salt
0.140	Banana chips
0.140	Soy sauce (soy & wheat)

0.140	Oysters, eastern, wild, cooked, moist heat
0.140	Chocolate-flavored hazelnut spread (No Trans Fat Data)
0.140	Acerola (West Indian cherry), raw (Missing Sugar and Vitamin Data)
0.131	Avg. Cheese
0.130	Anchovies, European, canned in oil, drained solids
0.130	Kale, boiled, drained, no salt
0.130	Lemon juice, raw
0.130	Corn chips, extruded, plain
0.120	Milk chocolate candies (No Trans Fat Data)
0.120	Ricotta cheese, whole milk (No Trans Fat Data)
0.120	Scallops (bay & sea), steamed
0.120	Cottage cheese, 1% milkfat (No Trans Fat Data)
0.120	Mushrooms, canned, drained solids
0.110	Lobster, northern, cooked in moist heat
0.110	Yogurt, regular low-fat, plain, 12 g protein per 8 oz
0.110	Tomato sauce, canned
0.110	Crayfish, mixed species, farmed, cooked in moist heat
0.110	Cream cheese (No Trans Fat Data)
0.109	Ginger, ground
0.106	Avg. Seafood
0.100	Peppers, sweet, green, raw
0.100	Ketchup
0.100	Parmesan cheese, grated (No Trans Fat Data)
0.100	Beef, eye of round, separable lean only, trimmed to 0" fat, all grades, roasted [cube steak]
0.100	Hamburger patty, 80/20 ground chuck beef, broiled
0.100	Oysters, eastern, wild, raw
0.100	Caraway seed
0.100	Celery seed
0.100	Cumin seed
0.100	Black pepper
0.100	Anise seed (Missing Sugar, Vitamin, O3FA data)
0.100	Macadamia nuts, dry roasted, with salt
0.100	Macadamia nuts, dry roasted, w/out salt
0.100	Provolone cheese (No Trans Fat Data)
0.090	Ice cream, soft-serve, french vanilla (No Trans Fat Data)

0.090	Mozzarella cheese, part skim (No Trans Fat Data)
0.090	Corned beef luncheon meat, beef, cured, canned (No Trans Fat Data)
0.090	Pumpkin/Squash Seeds, dry roasted, no salt (Missing Vitamin & Se Data)
0.090	Flounder (sole), cooked in dry heat
0.090	Swiss chard, boiled, drained, no salt
0.080	Spaghetti squash, winter, boiled w/out salt, drained
0.080	McDonald's barbeque sauce
0.080	American cheese, pasteurized, w/out disodium phosphate (No Trans Fat Data)
0.080	Mashed potatoes, home-prepared, whole milk & butter added
0.080	Teriyaki sauce, ready-to-serve
0.080	Chicken noodle soup prepared with equal volume water
0.070	Cucumber, raw w/ peel
0.070	T-bone steak, short loin, beef trimmed to 1/8" fat, all grades, broiled
0.070	Ground turkey, cooked
0.070	Bologna, chicken, pork, beef
0.070	Mustard, prepared, yellow
0.070	Mozzarella cheese, whole milk (No Trans Fat Data)
0.060	Blueberries, raw
0.060	Sweet potato, baked in skin, no salt
0.060	Hot Sauce (ready-to-serve, sauce, pepper or hot)
0.060	Turkey, fryer-roaster, breast meat only, roasted
0.060	Tilapia, cooked in dry heat
0.060	Red snapper, cooked, dry heat
0.060	Pastrami luncheon meat, beef, cured (No Trans Fat Data)
0.060	Hotdog, Oscar Mayer Wiener, beef frank (No Trans Fat Data)
0.060	Cinnamon
0.060	Bologna, lebanon, beef (No O3FA Data)
0.060	Swiss Cheese (No Trans Fat Data)
0.060	Oats, unenriched, boiled, w/out salt
0.053	Avg. Cased Meat
0.050	Raisins, seedless
0.050	Pineapple, canned, juice pack, drained
0.050	Black Tea, brewed with tap water
0.050	Milk, nonfat, added Vit A
0.050	Milk, nonfat, Ca fortified

0.050	Popcorn, caramel-coated without peanuts
0.050	Mayonnaise, soybean oil, w/ salt (salad dressing)
0.050	Ice creams, vanilla (No Trans Fat Data)
0.050	Avg. Lean Meat
0.050	Pepperoni, pork, beef
0.050	Sausage, Italian, pork, cooked (No Trans Fat Data)
0.050	Milk, lowfat, 1%, added Vit A
0.050	Milk, reduced fat, 2%, added Vit A
0.050	Milk, whole, 3.25% milkfat
0.040	Peaches, raw
0.040	Brown rice, long-grain, cooked
0.040	Light mayo (salad dressing)
0.040	Chicken, broilers or fryers, breast, meat only (no skin), roasted
0.040	Shrimp, mixed species, cooked in moist heat
0.040	Tuna fish, light, canned in water without salt, drained solids
0.040	Cherries, sweet, raw
0.033	Grits, corn, white, regular, quick, enriched, cooked with water, with salt
0.030	Garlic, raw
0.030	Apple, raw, with skin A343
0.030	Olives, pickled, canned or bottled, green
0.030	Margarine, industrial, non-dairy, cottonseed, soy oil (partially hydrogenated), for flaky pastries
0.030	Spam, Hormel (Missing Data)
0.030	Butter, salted (No Trans Fat Data)
0.020	Salami, dry or hard, pork (No Trans Fat Data)
0.020	Honey
0.020	Bacon (pork), cured, cooked, pan-fried
0.020	Salami, cooked, beef (No Trans Fat Data)
0.020	Grapes, red or green, European type such as Thompson seedless, raw
0.020	Swordfish, cooked in dry heat
0.020	Tuna fish, white, canned in water without salt, drained solids
0.017	Coffee, brewed from grounds w/ tap water, no sugar or cream (No O3FA Data)
0.010	Pickles, cucumber, dill or kosher dill
0.010	Swanson chicken broth, 99% Fat Free
0.010	Chamomile Tea (No O3FA & O6FA Data)

0.010	Apricot jam and preserves
0.010	Brown sugars
0.010	Margarine (vegetable oil spread, 70% fat, soybean & partially hydrogenated soybean, stick)
0.010	White rice, glutinous, cooked

Vitamin B12 (Cobalamin a.k.a. Cyanocobalamin)

Vitamin B12, ug/SS	Food
0.989	Clams, mixed species, cooked in moist heat
0.350	Oysters, eastern, wild, cooked, moist heat
0.195	Oysters, eastern, wild, raw
0.100	Wheaties, General Mills
0.097	Avg. Seafood
0.095	Corn Flakes, Kellogg's
0.095	Rice Krispies, Kellogg's
0.080	Frosted Flakes, Kellogg's
0.069	Cocoa Krispies, Kellogg's (No O3FA Data)
0.062	Cheerios, General Mills
0.060	Apple Jacks, Kellogg's
0.059	Lucky Charms, General Mills
0.056	Honey Smacks, Kellogg's
0.056	Golden Crisp, Post, Kraft
0.052	Cinnamon Toast Crunch cereal, ready-to-eat, General Mills
0.052	Honeycomb cereal, Post, Kraft (low data)
0.051	Kellogg's Raisin Bran
0.050	Bran Flakes, single brand
0.050	Cocoa Puffs, General Mills
0.049	Corn Pops, Kellogg's
0.048	Post Honey Bunches of Oats w/ Almonds (Missing Data)
0.047	Froot Loops, General Mills
0.035	Red snapper, cooked, dry heat
0.033	Swiss Cheese (No Trans Fat Data)
0.031	Lobster, northern, cooked in moist heat
0.031	Crayfish, mixed species, farmed, cooked in moist heat
0.031	Salami, cooked, beef (No Trans Fat Data)
0.031	Salmon, Atlantic, wild, cooked in dry heat
0.030	Tuna fish, light, canned in water without salt, drained solids
0.029	Bologna, lebanon, beef (No O3FA Data)
0.028	Salami, dry or hard, pork (No Trans Fat Data)
0.027	Hamburger patty, 80/20 ground chuck beef, broiled
0.026	Whiting, mixed species, cooked in dry heat

0.025	Flounder (sole), cooked in dry heat
0.023	Mozzarella cheese, whole milk (No Trans Fat Data)
0.023	Parmesan cheese, grated (No Trans Fat Data)
0.022	T-bone steak, short loin, beef trimmed to 1/8" fat, all grades, broiled
0.020	Swordfish, cooked in dry heat
0.019	Tilapia, cooked in dry heat
0.019	Pastrami luncheon meat, beef, cured (No Trans Fat Data)
0.018	Avg. Cased Meat
0.017	Pepperoni, pork, beef
0.016	Beef, eye of round, separable lean only, trimmed to 0" fat, all grades, roasted [cube steak]
0.016	Corned beef luncheon meat, beef, cured, canned (No Trans Fat Data)
0.016	Hotdog, Oscar Mayer Wiener, beef frank (No Trans Fat Data)
0.015	Shrimp, mixed species, cooked in moist heat
0.014	Provolone cheese (No Trans Fat Data)
0.014	Avg. Cheese
0.013	Bacon (pork), cured, cooked, pan-fried
0.013	Scallops (bay & sea), steamed
0.013	Sausage, Italian, pork, cooked (No Trans Fat Data)
0.012	Blue Cheese (No Trans Fat Data)
0.012	Tuna fish, white, canned in water without salt, drained solids
0.010	Beef sticks, smoked (No Trans Fat Data)
0.009	Anchovies, European, canned in oil, drained solids
0.008	Cheddar cheese (No Trans Fat Data)
0.008	Mozzarella cheese, part skim (No Trans Fat Data)
0.008	Egg, whole, cooked, scrambled
0.008	Milk chocolate candies (No Trans Fat Data)
0.007	Avg. Lean Meat
0.007	American cheese, pasteurized, w/out disodium phosphate (No Trans Fat Data)
0.006	Cottage cheese, 1% milkfat (No Trans Fat Data)
0.006	Pork-skins, plain
0.006	Pork tenderloin lean, roasted, URMIS 3358
0.006	Bologna, chicken, pork, beef
0.006	Slice of pizza, fast food, pizza chain, 14", cheese topping, regular crust (No Trans Fat Data)
0.006	Yogurt, regular low-fat, plain, 12 g protein per 8 oz

0.005	Milk, nonfat, added Vit A
0.005	Cheese-flavor puffs or twists, corn-based
0.005	Ice cream, soft-serve, french vanilla (No Trans Fat Data)
0.005	Milk, lowfat, 1%, added Vit A
0.005	Milk, reduced fat, 2%, added Vit A
0.005	Milk, whole, 3.25% milkfat
0.004	Tortilla chips, plain, white corn
0.004	Ice creams, vanilla (No Trans Fat Data)
0.004	Turkey, fryer-roaster, breast meat only, roasted
0.004	Milk, nonfat, Ca fortified
0.004	Chicken, broilers or fryers, breast, meat only (no skin), roasted
0.003	Turkey, stuffing, mashed potatoes w/ gravy, assorted vegetables, frozen, microwaved
0.003	Mayonnaise, soybean oil, w/ salt (salad dressing)
0.003	Ricotta cheese, whole milk (No Trans Fat Data)
0.003	Ground turkey, cooked
0.003	Chocolate-flavored hazelnut spread (No Trans Fat Data)
0.003	Ramen noodle soup, chicken flavor, dry
0.003	Cream cheese (No Trans Fat Data)
0.002	Swanson chicken broth, 99% Fat Free
0.002	Margarine, industrial, non-dairy, cottonseed, soy oil (partially hydrogenated), for flaky pastries
0.002	Dark chocolate candies, 60-69% cacao solids (Missing Vitamin Data)
0.002	Candy bar, Snickers (King Size)
0.002	Butter, salted (No Trans Fat Data)
0.001	Mushrooms, portabella, raw
0.001	Cake, snack cakes, crème-filled, chocolate with frosting
0.001	Egg noodles, cooked, enriched

Choline

Choline, mg/SS	Food
1.900	Egg, whole, cooked, scrambled
1.640	Pork-skins, plain
1.310	Bacon (pork), cured, cooked, pan-fried
1.230	Mustard seed, yellow
1.120	Beef, eye of round, separable lean only, trimmed to 0" fat, all grades, roasted [cube steak]
0.971	Cilantro, dried (No O3FA Data)
0.971	Parsley, dried (Missing O3FA Data)
0.927	T-bone steak, short loin, beef trimmed to 1/8" fat, all grades, broiled
0.926	Avg. Lean Meat
0.892	Corned beef luncheon meat, beef, cured, canned (No Trans Fat Data)
0.889	Pork tenderloin lean, roasted, URMIS 3358
0.850	Chicken, broilers or fryers, breast, meat only (no skin), roasted
0.850	Anchovies, European, canned in oil, drained solids
0.844	Turkey, fryer-roaster, breast meat only, roasted
0.817	Avg. Seafood
0.816	Pastrami luncheon meat, beef, cured (No Trans Fat Data)
0.811	Flounder (sole), cooked in dry heat
0.810	Scallops (bay & sea), steamed
0.810	Whiting, mixed species, cooked in dry heat
0.809	Shrimp, mixed species, cooked in moist heat
0.808	Hamburger patty, 80/20 ground chuck beef, broiled
0.807	Lobster, northern, cooked in moist heat
0.787	Flaxseed
0.782	Sausage, Italian, pork, cooked (No Trans Fat Data)
0.771	Pepperoni, pork, beef
0.750	Ground turkey, cooked
0.714	Pistachio nuts, dry roasted, no salt
0.665	Chili powder
0.659	Peanut butter, smooth, USDA Commodity
0.649	Oysters, eastern, wild, raw
0.642	Curry powder
0.627	Bologna, lebanon, beef (No O3FA Data)
0.610	Cashews, dry roasted, no salt

0.591	Bologna, chicken, pork, beef
0.575	Salami, cooked, beef (No Trans Fat Data)
0.563	Edamame beans, frozen, prepared
0.553	Avg. Cased Meat
0.553	Peanuts, dry roasted, no salt, all types
0.551	Sunflower Seeds, hulled, dry roased, no salt
0.549	Basil, dried
0.529	Avg. Nuts
0.521	Almonds, USDA A256, A264
0.515	Paprika
0.498	Lard (No Trans Fat Data)
0.492	Turmeric, ground
0.475	Soybeans green, boiled, drained, no salt
0.461	Milk chocolate candies (No Trans Fat Data)
0.452	Cauliflower, raw
0.446	Macadamia nuts, dry roasted, with salt
0.446	Macadamia nuts, dry roasted, w/out salt
0.444	Avg. Spice
0.441	Lima beans, immature, boiled, drained, no salt
0.436	Marjoram, dried
0.436	Sage, ground
0.436	Thyme, dried
0.436	Avg. Herbs
0.428	Chick peas (garbanzo, bengal gram), mature seeds, boiled, no salt
0.400	Broccoli, boiled, drained, no salt
0.395	Potato flour
0.392	Walnuts, USDA A259, A257
0.385	Candy bar, Snickers (King Size)
0.374	Cloves, ground
0.368	Mushrooms, shiitake, cooked, no salt
0.353	Pinto beans, boiled, no salt, mature
0.338	Kellogg's Nutri-Grain Cereal Bars, fruit-filled
0.333	Avg. Beans & Lentils
0.329	Wheaties, General Mills
0.327	Soy sauce, low sodium (soy & wheat)
0.327	Lentils, mature seeds, boiled, no salt

0.326	Chick peas (garbanzo, bengal gram), mature seeds, canned
0.323	Oregano, dried
0.321	Rice cakes, brown rice, plain
0.312	Whole wheat flour
0.305	Kidney beans, red, boiled, no salt, mature seeds
0.304	Rye
0.295	Pretzels, hard, plain, salted
0.291	Corn, sweet, yellow, boiled, drained, no salt
0.290	Kellogg's Raisin Bran
0.288	Brazil nuts, dried, unblanched
0.287	Swiss chard, boiled, drained, no salt
0.278	Hummus, home prepared
0.276	Bran Flakes, single brand
0.275	Peas, frozen, boiled, drained, no salt
0.272	Cream cheese (No Trans Fat Data)
0.265	Whole wheat bread, commecially prepared
0.265	Whole wheat bread, prepared from recipe
0.265	Whole wheat pita bread
0.262	Cheerios, General Mills
0.260	Ice creams, vanilla (No Trans Fat Data)
0.260	Ice cream, soft-serve, french vanilla (No Trans Fat Data)
0.257	Egg noodles, cooked, enriched
0.247	Caraway seed
0.247	Celery seed
0.247	Cumin seed
0.235	Popcorn, caramel-coated without peanuts
0.232	Garlic, raw
0.231	Puffed Wheat, Quaker
0.224	Mustard, prepared, yellow
0.218	Mayonnaise, soybean oil, w/ salt (salad dressing)
0.213	Banana chips
0.212	Mushrooms, portabella, raw
0.212	Popcorn, air-popped
0.206	Cake, snack cakes, crème-filled, chocolate with frosting
0.203	Cabbage, boiled, drained, no salt
0.200	Honey Smacks, Kellogg's

0.199	Mushrooms, boiled, drained, no salt
0.199	Mushrooms, canned, drained solids
0.197	Spinach, boiled, drained, no salt
0.195	Teriyaki sauce, ready-to-serve
0.194	Tortilla chips, plain, white corn
0.189	Potato, red, baked, flesh & skin
0.188	Butter, salted (No Trans Fat Data)
0.187	Avg. Leafy Green Vegetables
0.187	Wheat dinner rolls
0.183	Soy sauce (soy & wheat)
0.177	Milk, lowfat, 1%, added Vit A
0.177	Pretzels, soft
0.176	Chocolate-flavored hazelnut spread (No Trans Fat Data)
0.175	Ricotta cheese, whole milk (No Trans Fat Data)
0.175	Cottage cheese, 1% milkfat (No Trans Fat Data)
0.173	Avg. Cheese
0.171	Turkey, stuffing, mashed potatoes w/ gravy, assorted vegetables, frozen, microwaved
0.170	Sesame sticks, wheat-based, salted
0.169	Snap (green string) beans, boiled, drained, no salt
0.167	Granola bar, soft, uncoated, chocolate chip
0.165	Cheddar cheese (No Trans Fat Data)
0.164	Slice of pizza, fast food, pizza chain, 14", cheese topping, regular crust (No Trans Fat Data)
0.164	Milk, reduced fat, 2%, added Vit A
0.162	Lucky Charms, General Mills
0.160	Milk, nonfat, Ca fortified
0.160	Asparagus, raw
0.156	Milk, nonfat, added Vit A
0.155	Swiss Cheese (No Trans Fat Data)
0.154	Parmesan cheese, grated (No Trans Fat Data)
0.154	Blue Cheese (No Trans Fat Data)
0.154	Mozzarella cheese, part skim (No Trans Fat Data)
0.154	Provolone cheese (No Trans Fat Data)
0.154	Mozzarella cheese, whole milk (No Trans Fat Data)
0.152	Yogurt, regular low-fat, plain, 12 g protein per 8 oz
0.150	Potato, Russet, baked, flesh & skin

0.148	FritoLay Sun Chips, Multi-grain snack, original flavor
0.148	Potato, baked, flesh & skin, no salt
0.147	Peanut Butter Cap'n Crunch, Quaker
0.146	White bread, commercially prepared (inlcudes soft crumbs)
0.146	Roll, hard, kaiser
0.146	White pita bread, enriched
0.143	Milk, whole, 3.25% milkfat
0.142	Olives, pickled, canned or bottled, green
0.142	Avocado, raw, commercial varieties
0.141	Cap'n Crunch with Crunch Berries, Quaker
0.139	Popcorn, regular butter flavor, microwave, made w/ partially hydrogenated oil (Missing Fats Data)
0.131	Sweet potato, baked in skin, no salt
0.130	Popcorn, microwave, 94% fat free
0.125	Ketchup
0.123	Raspberries, raw
0.121	Corn chips, extruded, plain
0.121	Pak-choi, boiled, drained, no salt
0.121	Potato chips, plain, salted
0.121	Coconut meat, raw
0.116	Cheese-flavor puffs or twists, corn-based
0.115	Ginger, ground
0.114	Basil, fresh
0.113	Avg. Vegetables
0.113	Black pepper
0.112	Millet, cooked
0.111	Raisins, seedless
0.110	Cinnamon
0.108	Matzo crackers, plain
0.105	Froot Loops, General Mills
0.104	White flour, white, all-purpose, enriched, bleached
0.102	Wild rice, cooked
0.099	Tomato sauce, canned
0.099	Romaine or cos lettuce
0.099	Cap'n Crunch, Quaker
0.098	Banana, raw

0.094	Eggplant, boiled, drained, no salt
0.094	Cinnamon Toast Crunch cereal, ready-to-eat, General Mills
0.094	Zucchini, summer squash, w/ skin, boiled w/out salt, drained
0.092	Brown rice, long-grain, cooked
0.088	Carrots, raw, USDA A099
0.088	Poppy seed
0.088	Nutmeg, ground (Missing O3FA Data)
0.087	Cocoa Krispies, Kellogg's (No O3FA Data)
0.086	Orange, raw, all commercial varieties
0.084	Rice Krispies, Kellogg's
0.076	Cantaloupe, raw
0.076	Pomegranate, raw
0.076	Cocoa Puffs, General Mills
0.076	Mangos, raw
0.075	Beets, canned, drained solids
0.075	Spaghetti squash, winter, boiled w/out salt, drained
0.070	Avg. Fruit
0.067	Tomatoes, raw, red, ripe
0.067	Iceberg lettuce
0.065	Horseradish, prepared
0.065	Radishes, raw
0.064	Spaghetti, cooked, enriched w/out added salt, no sauce
0.061	Onion, raw
0.061	Peaches, raw
0.061	Cherries, sweet, raw
0.061	Papayas, raw
0.060	Beets, raw
0.060	Cucumber, raw w/ peel
0.060	Blueberries, raw
0.057	Strawberries, raw
0.056	Grapes, red or green, European type such as Thompson seedless, raw
0.056	Peppers, sweet, red, raw
0.055	Pineapple, canned, juice pack, drained
0.055	Pineapple, raw, all varieties
0.055	Peppers, sweet, green, raw
0.055	Chicken noodle soup prepared with equal volume water

0.051	Lemon juice, raw
0.039	Corn Flakes, Kellogg's
0.034	Pickles, cucumber, dill or kosher dill
0.034	Apple, raw, with skin A343
0.033	Apple Jacks, Kellogg's
0.032	Grape Juice, canned or bottled, unsweetened
0.030	Corn Pops, Kellogg's
0.030	Frosted Flakes, Kellogg's
0.023	Brown sugars
0.023	Coffee, brewed from grounds w/ tap water, no sugar or cream (No O3FA Data)
0.022	Honey
0.021	White rice, glutinous, cooked
0.021	White rice, long-grain, pre-cooked or instant, prepared (Missing O3FA Data)
0.021	White rice, long-grain, regular, cooked
0.021	Parboiled rice, white, long-grain, enriched, cooked
0.018	Apple Juice, canned or bottled, unsweetened
0.016	Syrups, maple
0.011	Cranberry juice cocktail, bottled
0.004	Sprite
0.004	Apricot jam and preserves
0.004	Corn starch (Missing O3FA Data)
0.004	Kale, boiled, drained, no salt
0.004	Chamomile Tea (No O3FA & O6FA Data)
0.004	Black Tea, brewed with tap water
0.003	Coconut oil (Missing Trans Fat & O3FA Data)
0.003	Olive oil (Missing Trans Fat Data)
0.002	Shortening, industrial, soy (partially hydrogenated) for baking & confections (Missing O3FA Data)
0.002	Vegetable shortening, household, composite
0.002	Sesame oil (Missing Trans Fat Data)
0.002	Canola oil (vegetable oil), low erucic acid rapeseed oil
0.002	Cottonseed (vegetable oil), salad or cooking (Missing Trans Fat Data)
0.002	Corn oil (vegetable oil), industrial and retail, all purpose salad or cooking
0.002	Soybean oil, salad or cooking (Missing Phytosterol Data)

0.002	Shortening, vegetable, industrial, soy (partially hydrogenated), all purpose
0.001	Peanut oil, salad or cooking (No Trans Fat or O3FA Data)

Betaine

Betaine, mg/SS	Food
5.772	Spinach, boiled, drained, no salt
2.554	Beets, canned, drained solids
1.990	Wheaties, General Mills
1.287	Beets, raw
0.826	Avg. Leafy Green Vegetables
0.728	Whole wheat flour
0.703	White flour, white, all-purpose, enriched, bleached
0.680	Spaghetti, cooked, enriched w/out added salt, no sauce
0.500	Pretzels, hard, plain, salted
0.391	FritoLay Sun Chips, Multi-grain snack, original flavor
0.364	Cake, snack cakes, crème-filled, chocolate with frosting
0.347	Cheerios, General Mills
0.346	Sweet potato, baked in skin, no salt
0.298	Soy sauce (soy & wheat)
0.288	Curry powder
0.278	Slice of pizza, fast food, pizza chain, 14", cheese topping, regular crust (No Trans Fat Data)
0.216	Granola bar, soft, uncoated, chocolate chip
0.192	Egg noodles, cooked, enriched
0.161	Basil, dried
0.147	Beef, eye of round, separable lean only, trimmed to 0" fat, all grades, roasted [cube steak]
0.131	Avg. Vegetables
0.130	Avg. Herbs
0.122	T-bone steak, short loin, beef trimmed to 1/8" fat, all grades, broiled
0.117	Corned beef luncheon meat, beef, cured, canned (No Trans Fat Data)
0.107	Pastrami luncheon meat, beef, cured (No Trans Fat Data)
0.098	Oregano, dried
0.097	Turmeric, ground
0.089	Black pepper
0.081	Avg. Spice
0.080	Hamburger patty, 80/20 ground chuck beef, broiled
0.078	Avg. Lean Meat
0.071	Paprika

0.068	Bologna, lebanon, beef (No O3FA Data)
0.064	Turkey, stuffing, mashed potatoes w/ gravy, assorted vegetables, frozen, microwaved
0.062	Chicken, broilers or fryers, breast, meat only (no skin), roasted
0.061	Mushrooms, portabella, raw
0.061	Turkey, fryer-roaster, breast meat only, roasted
0.055	Ground turkey, cooked
0.045	Avg. Cased Meat
0.045	Edamame beans, frozen, prepared
0.043	Pork tenderloin lean, roasted, URMIS 3358
0.042	Bacon (pork), cured, cooked, pan-fried
0.042	Bologna, chicken, pork, beef
0.042	Sausage, Italian, pork, cooked (No Trans Fat Data)
0.039	Cinnamon
0.031	Oats, unenriched, boiled, w/out salt
0.031	Flaxseed
0.028	Pepperoni, pork, beef
0.027	Chili powder
0.026	Milk chocolate candies (No Trans Fat Data)
0.026	Salami, cooked, beef (No Trans Fat Data)
0.019	Milk, nonfat, added Vit A
0.019	Mustard seed, yellow
0.017	Honey
0.017	Parsley, dried (Missing O3FA Data)
0.014	Cloves, ground
0.013	Cocoa Krispies, Kellogg's (No O3FA Data)
0.010	Ginger, ground
0.009	Milk, reduced fat, 2%, added Vit A
0.009	Poppy seed
0.009	Yogurt, regular low-fat, plain, 12 g protein per 8 oz
0.009	Candy bar, Snickers (King Size)
0.008	Tomato sauce, canned
0.008	Raspberries, raw
0.008	Pistachio nuts, dry roasted, no salt
0.008	Popcorn, air-popped
0.007	Corn Flakes, Kellogg's

0.007	Avocado, raw, commercial varieties
0.007	Avg. Beans & Lentils
0.007	Cream cheese (No Trans Fat Data)
0.007	Cheddar cheese (No Trans Fat Data)
0.007	Avg. Cheese
0.006	Milk, lowfat, 1%, added Vit A
0.006	Milk, whole, 3.25% milkfat
0.006	Swiss Cheese (No Trans Fat Data)
0.006	Egg, whole, cooked, scrambled
0.006	Asparagus, raw
0.005	Brown rice, long-grain, cooked
0.005	Cheese-flavor puffs or twists, corn-based
0.005	Rice Krispies, Kellogg's
0.005	Almonds, USDA A256, A264
0.005	Avg. Nuts
0.004	Tortilla chips, plain, white corn
0.004	Basil, fresh
0.004	Carrots, raw, USDA A099
0.004	Peanut butter, smooth, USDA Commodity
0.004	Brazil nuts, dried, unblanched
0.003	Walnuts, USDA A259, A257
0.003	White rice, long-grain, regular, cooked
0.003	Butter, salted (No Trans Fat Data)
0.003	Kale, boiled, drained, no salt
0.003	Macadamia nuts, dry roasted, with salt
0.003	Macadamia nuts, dry roasted, w/out salt
0.003	Raisins, seedless
0.003	Cabbage, boiled, drained, no salt
0.003	Popcorn, microwave, 94% fat free
0.003	Popcorn, regular butter flavor, microwave, made w/ partially hydrogenated oil (Missing Fats Data)
0.003	Peaches, raw
0.003	Zucchini, summer squash, w/ skin, boiled w/out salt, drained
0.002	Avg. Fruit
0.002	Potato chips, plain, salted
0.002	Ketchup

0.002	Mustard, prepared, yellow
0.002	Potato, baked, flesh & skin, no salt
0.002	Potato, red, baked, flesh & skin
0.002	Potato, Russet, baked, flesh & skin
0.002	Blueberries, raw
0.002	Grape Juice, canned or bottled, unsweetened
0.002	Strawberries, raw
0.002	Pak-choi, boiled, drained, no salt
0.001	Grapes, red or green, European type such as Thompson seedless, raw
0.001	Onion, raw
0.001	Pineapple, raw, all varieties
0.001	Peas, frozen, boiled, drained, no salt
0.001	Cranberry juice cocktail, bottled
0.001	Pinto beans, boiled, no salt, mature
0.001	Apple Juice, canned or bottled, unsweetened
0.001	Swiss chard, boiled, drained, no salt
0.001	Broccoli, boiled, drained, no salt
0.001	Corn chips, extruded, plain
0.001	Iceberg lettuce
0.001	Romaine or cos lettuce
0.001	Cucumber, raw w/ peel
0.001	Cantaloupe, raw
0.001	Olive oil (Missing Trans Fat Data)
0.001	Brown sugars
0.001	Apple, raw, with skin A343
0.001	Radishes, raw
0.001	Snap (green string) beans, boiled, drained, no salt
0.001	Banana, raw
0.001	Tomatoes, raw, red, ripe
0.001	Peppers, sweet, green, raw
0.001	Peppers, sweet, red, raw

Calcium

Calcium, mg/SS	Food
21.130	Basil, dried
19.900	Marjoram, dried
18.900	Thyme, dried
18.442	Avg. Herbs
17.840	Dill weed, dried (Missing Data)
17.670	Celery seed
16.520	Sage, ground
15.760	Oregano, dried
14.680	Parsley, dried (Missing O3FA Data)
14.380	Poppy seed
12.800	Rosemary, dried (Missing Data)
12.460	Cilantro, dried (No O3FA Data)
11.960	Fennel seed (Missing Vitamin & O3FA Data)
11.390	Tarragon, dried (Missing Data)
11.090	Parmesan cheese, grated (No Trans Fat Data)
10.020	Cinnamon
9.310	Cumin seed
8.340	Bay leaf (Missing Data)
7.909	Swiss Cheese (No Trans Fat Data)
7.820	Mozzarella cheese, part skim (No Trans Fat Data)
7.561	Provolone cheese (No Trans Fat Data)
7.212	Cheddar cheese (No Trans Fat Data)
7.090	Coriander seed (Missing Data)
6.890	Caraway seed
6.610	Allspice (Missing Data)
6.463	Avg. Spice
6.460	Cloves, ground
6.460	Anise seed (Missing Sugar, Vitamin, O3FA data)
6.310	Chia seeds, dried (Missing Sugar and Vitamin Data)
6.160	American cheese, pasteurized, w/out disodium phosphate (No Trans Fat Data)
5.924	Avg. Cheese
5.410	Kellogg's Nutri-Grain Cereal Bars, fruit-filled
5.280	Blue Cheese (No Trans Fat Data)

5.210	Mustard seed, yellow
5.054	Mozzarella cheese, whole milk (No Trans Fat Data)
4.780	Curry powder
4.660	Velveeta cheese, Kraft, pasteurized spread (Missing Data)
4.510	Cinnamon Toast Crunch cereal, ready-to-eat, General Mills
4.370	Black pepper
4.080	Cheerios, General Mills
4.050	Thyme, fresh (Missing Data)
3.990	Lucky Charms, General Mills
3.830	Cardamom (Missing Data)
3.330	Cocoa Puffs, General Mills
3.170	Rosemarry, fresh (Missing Data)
2.780	Chili powder
2.643	Almonds, USDA A256, A264
2.550	Flaxseed
2.520	Mace, ground (Missing Data)
2.500	Whey protein powder (Low Data)
2.320	Anchovies, European, canned in oil, drained solids
2.070	Ricotta cheese, whole milk (No Trans Fat Data)
2.040	Milk, nonfat, Ca fortified
1.990	Spearmint, fresh (Missing Data)
1.887	Milk chocolate candies (No Trans Fat Data)
1.840	Nutmeg, ground (Missing O3FA Data)
1.830	Turmeric, ground
1.829	Yogurt, regular low-fat, plain, 12 g protein per 8 oz
1.809	Garlic, raw
1.770	Paprika
1.770	Basil, fresh
1.767	Slice of pizza, fast food, pizza chain, 14", cheese topping, regular crust (No Trans Fat Data)
1.760	Wheat dinner rolls
1.760	Fenugreek seed (Missing Vitamin & O3, 6FA Data)
1.740	Tortilla chips, plain, white corn
1.700	Sesame sticks, wheat-based, salted
1.641	Corn chips, extruded, plain
1.602	Brazil nuts, dried, unblanched

1.540	Ritz Crackers, Nabisco (Missing Vitamin Data)
1.510	White bread, commercially prepared (inlcudes soft crumbs)
1.401	Soybeans (aka soy nuts) mature, dry roasted (Missing Sugar and Vitamin Data)
1.361	Spinach, boiled, drained, no salt
1.320	Kraft macaroni & cheese dinner, original, unprepared (Missing Data)
1.310	Ice cream, soft-serve, french vanilla (No Trans Fat Data)
1.280	Ice creams, vanilla (No Trans Fat Data)
1.249	Milk, nonfat, added Vit A
1.189	Milk, lowfat, 1%, added Vit A
1.176	Greek yogurt
1.172	Milk, reduced fat, 2%, added Vit A
1.160	Cake, snack cakes, crème-filled, chocolate with frosting
1.150	Scallops (bay & sea), steamed
1.131	Milk, whole, 3.25% milkfat
1.110	Saffron (Missing Data)
1.098	Pistachio nuts, dry roasted, no salt
1.080	Chocolate-flavored hazelnut spread (No Trans Fat Data)
1.070	Whole wheat bread, commecially prepared
1.017	Soybeans green, boiled, drained, no salt
0.983	Walnuts, USDA A259, A257
0.978	Cream cheese (No Trans Fat Data)
0.950	Roll, hard, kaiser
0.948	Avg. Nuts
0.940	Tortilla chips, plain, yellow corn (Missing Vitamin Data)
0.929	Pak-choi, boiled, drained, no salt
0.929	Candy bar, Snickers (King Size)
0.920	Clams, mixed species, cooked in moist heat
0.920	Bologna, chicken, pork, beef
0.900	Oysters, eastern, wild, cooked, moist heat
0.860	White pita bread, enriched
0.832	Brown sugars
0.780	Froot Loops, General Mills
0.741	Weight Watchers Smart Ones Chicken Enchiladas Suiza, Sour Cream w/ Cheese frozen entrée (Missing Data)
0.740	Bagel, plain, unenriched w/ calcium propionate, onion, poppy, sesame (no cream cheese)

0.738	Instant Oatmeal, Quaker, apples & cinnamon prepared w/ boiling water
0.720	Kale, boiled, drained, no salt
0.720	Pecans, dry roasted, no salt
0.710	Egg, whole, cooked, scrambled
0.700	Macadamia nuts, dry roasted, with salt
0.700	Macadamia nuts, dry roasted, w/out salt
0.700	Sunflower Seeds, hulled, dry roased, no salt
0.685	Avg. Leafy Green Vegetables
0.680	Beef sticks, smoked (No Trans Fat Data)
0.671	Syrups, maple
0.670	Wheaties, General Mills
0.667	Greek style yogurt 150g=2/3 cup (Missing Data)
0.660	Margarine, industrial, non-dairy, cottonseed, soy oil (partially hydrogenated), for flaky pastries
0.650	Potato flour
0.639	Cream of Wheat, instant, prepared with water and salt
0.630	Edamame beans, frozen, prepared
0.620	Whiting, mixed species, cooked in dry heat
0.620	Dark chocolate candies, 60-69% cacao solids (Missing Vitamin Data)
0.611	Cottage cheese, 1% milkfat (No Trans Fat Data)
0.610	Lobster, northern, cooked in moist heat
0.580	Cheese-flavor puffs or twists, corn-based
0.578	Mustard, prepared, yellow
0.577	Swiss chard, boiled, drained, no salt
0.560	Horseradish, prepared
0.560	Bran Flakes, single brand
0.550	Pumpkin/Squash Seeds, dry roasted, no salt (Missing Vitamin & Se Data)
0.545	Avg. Seafood
0.540	Oats
0.540	Peanuts, dry roasted, no salt, all types
0.539	Peanut butter, smooth, USDA Commodity
0.520	Olives, pickled, canned or bottled, green
0.510	Crayfish, mixed species, farmed, cooked in moist heat
0.500	Raisins, seedless
0.492	Hummus, home prepared

0.490	Chick peas (garbanzo, bengal gram), mature seeds, boiled, no salt
0.480	Cabbage, boiled, drained, no salt
0.470	Kellogg's Raisin Bran
0.460	Pinto beans, boiled, no salt, mature
0.452	Oysters, eastern, wild, raw
0.450	Cashews, dry roasted, no salt
0.440	Snap (green string) beans, boiled, drained, no salt
0.431	Avg. Beans & Lentils
0.430	Popcorn, caramel-coated without peanuts
0.420	Pickles, cucumber, dill or kosher dill
0.410	Granola bar, soft, uncoated, chocolate chip
0.410	Butternut squash, winter, baked w/out salt, sugar or butter
0.409	Orange, raw, all commercial varieties
0.400	Broccoli, boiled, drained, no salt
0.400	Red snapper, cooked, dry heat
0.390	Shrimp, mixed species, cooked in moist heat
0.380	Sweet potato, baked in skin, no salt
0.370	Post Honey Bunches of Oats w/ Almonds (Missing Data)
0.350	Black beans, mature seeds, canned
0.340	Whole wheat flour
0.330	Rye
0.330	Romaine or cos lettuce
0.330	Whole wheat bread, prepared from recipe
0.330	Barley (hulled)
0.330	Carrots, raw, USDA A099
0.325	Ginger, ground
0.320	Chick peas (garbanzo, bengal gram), mature seeds, canned
0.320	Lima beans, immature, boiled, drained, no salt
0.300	Pork-skins, plain
0.280	Kidney beans, red, boiled, no salt, mature seeds
0.280	Pretzels, hard, whole-wheat (Missing Sugar Data)
0.270	Turkey, stuffing, mashed potatoes w/ gravy, assorted vegetables, frozen, microwaved
0.270	Ramen noodle soup, chicken flavor, dry
0.250	Radishes, raw
0.250	Teriyaki sauce, ready-to-serve

0.250	Ground turkey, cooked
0.250	Raspberries, raw
0.240	Asparagus, raw
0.240	Potato chips, plain, salted
0.240	Butter, salted (No Trans Fat Data)
0.240	Salt (table salt)
0.240	Papayas, raw
0.240	Puffed Wheat, Quaker
0.240	Honey Smacks, Kellogg's
0.240	Hamburger patty, 80/20 ground chuck beef, broiled
0.240	Mashed potatoes, home-prepared, whole milk & butter added
0.240	Peas, frozen, boiled, drained, no salt
0.233	Avg. Cased Meat
0.230	Pretzels, soft
0.230	Onion, raw
0.220	Cauliflower, raw
0.220	Pepperoni, pork, beef
0.210	Spaghetti squash, winter, boiled w/out salt, drained
0.210	Sausage, Italian, pork, cooked (No Trans Fat Data)
0.200	FritoLay Sun Chips, Multi-grain snack, original flavor
0.200	Apricot jam and preserves
0.200	Popcorn, regular butter flavor, microwave, made w/ partially hydrogenated oil (Missing Fats Data)
0.200	Bologna, lebanon, beef (No O3FA Data)
0.190	Lentils, mature seeds, boiled, no salt
0.190	Parboiled rice, white, long-grain, enriched, cooked
0.190	Soy sauce (soy & wheat)
0.180	Flounder (sole), cooked in dry heat
0.180	Ketchup
0.180	Iceberg lettuce
0.180	Banana chips
0.180	Pretzels, hard, plain, salted
0.180	Banquest Hearty Ones Salisbury Steak Dinner w/ Gravy, Mashed Potatoes and Corn in Seasoned Sauce, frozen meal(Missing Data)
0.180	Potato, Russet, baked, flesh & skin
0.178	Avg. Vegetables
0.170	Quinoa, cooked

0.170	Soy sauce, low sodium (soy & wheat)
0.170	McDonald's French Fries
0.170	Corn Pops, Kellogg's
0.170	Cocoa Krispies, Kellogg's (No O3FA Data)
0.170	Honeycomb cereal, Post, Kraft (low data)
0.160	Beets, raw
0.160	Pineapple, canned, juice pack, drained
0.160	Cucumber, raw w/ peel
0.160	Strawberries, raw
0.150	Salmon, Atlantic, wild, cooked in dry heat
0.150	Whole wheat pita bread
0.150	Golden Crisp, Post, Kraft
0.150	Chicken, broilers or fryers, breast, meat only (no skin), roasted
0.150	Beets, canned, drained solids
0.150	Banquet chicken pot pie, frozen entrée (Missing Data)
0.150	Potato, baked, flesh & skin, no salt
0.150	White flour, white, all-purpose, enriched, bleached
0.140	Tuna fish, white, canned in water without salt, drained solids
0.140	Water, bottled, Perrier
0.140	Coconut meat, raw
0.140	Popcorn, microwave, 94% fat free
0.140	Cap'n Crunch with Crunch Berries, Quaker
0.140	Tilapia, cooked in dry heat
0.140	Spam, Hormel (Missing Data)
0.138	Avg. Fruit
0.130	Pineapple, raw, all varieties
0.130	Tomato sauce, canned
0.130	Salami, dry or hard, pork (No Trans Fat Data)
0.130	Zucchini, summer squash, w/ skin, boiled w/out salt, drained
0.130	Matzo crackers, plain
0.130	Cherries, sweet, raw
0.120	Egg noodles, cooked, enriched
0.120	Turkey, fryer-roaster, breast meat only, roasted
0.120	Bacon (pork), cured, cooked, pan-fried
0.120	Corned beef luncheon meat, beef, cured, canned (No Trans Fat Data)
0.120	Salsa, USDA Commodity (Missing Sugar and Vitamin Data)

0.120	Acerola (West Indian cherry), raw (Missing Sugar and Vitamin Data)
0.120	Avocado, raw, commercial varieties
0.110	Tuna fish, light, canned in water without salt, drained solids
0.110	Mushrooms, canned, drained solids
0.110	Rice cakes, brown rice, plain
0.110	McDonald's barbeque sauce
0.110	Apple Jacks, Kellogg's
0.110	Cap'n Crunch, Quaker
0.110	Grape Juice, canned or bottled, unsweetened
0.100	Pomegranate, raw
0.100	Mangos, raw
0.100	Tomatoes, raw, red, ripe
0.100	Peppers, sweet, green, raw
0.100	White rice, long-grain, regular, cooked
0.100	Brown rice, long-grain, cooked
0.100	Pastrami luncheon meat, beef, cured (No Trans Fat Data)
0.100	Hotdog, Oscar Mayer Wiener, beef frank (No Trans Fat Data)
0.100	Grapes, red or green, European type such as Thompson seedless, raw
0.098	Avg. Lean Meat
0.090	Cantaloupe, raw
0.090	Oats, unenriched, boiled, w/out salt
0.090	McDonald's spicy buffalo sauce
0.090	Peanut Butter Cap'n Crunch, Quaker
0.090	Potato, red, baked, flesh & skin
0.080	Apple Juice, canned or bottled, unsweetened
0.080	T-bone steak, short loin, beef trimmed to 1/8" fat, all grades, broiled
0.080	Mushrooms, portabella, raw
0.080	Hot Sauce (ready-to-serve, sauce, pepper or hot)
0.080	Light mayo (salad dressing)
0.080	White rice, long-grain, pre-cooked or instant, prepared (Missing O3FA Data)
0.080	New England clam chowder, Campbell's Select (Missing Data)
0.070	Lemon juice, raw
0.070	Spaghetti, cooked, enriched w/out added salt, no sauce
0.070	Popcorn, air-popped
0.070	Mayonnaise, soybean oil, w/ salt (salad dressing)

0.070	Rice Krispies, Kellogg's
0.070	Margarine (vegetable oil spread, 70% fat, soybean & partially hydrogenated soybean, stick)
0.070	Peppers, sweet, red, raw
0.060	Swordfish, cooked in dry heat
0.060	Mushrooms, boiled, drained, no salt
0.060	Apple, raw, with skin A343
0.060	Chicken noodle soup prepared with equal volume water
0.060	Blueberries, raw
0.060	Peaches, raw
0.060	Eggplant, boiled, drained, no salt
0.060	Beef, eye of round, separable lean only, trimmed to 0" fat, all grades, roasted [cube steak]
0.060	Pork tenderloin lean, roasted, URMIS 3358
0.060	Salami, cooked, beef (No Trans Fat Data)
0.060	Honey
0.050	Banana, raw
0.040	Swanson chicken broth, 99% Fat Free
0.040	Corn Flakes, Kellogg's
0.040	Rice noodles, cooked (Missing Sugar & Unsaturated Fat Data)
0.030	Mushrooms, shiitake, cooked, no salt
0.030	Grits, corn, white, regular, quick, enriched, cooked with water, with salt
0.030	Cranberry juice cocktail, bottled
0.030	Frosted Flakes, Kellogg's
0.030	Water, tap, drinking
0.030	Ginger Ale
0.030	Millet, cooked
0.030	Corn, sweet, yellow, boiled, drained, no salt
0.030	Wild rice, cooked
0.020	Corn starch (Missing O3FA Data)
0.020	White rice, glutinous, cooked
0.020	Sprite
0.020	Chamomile Tea (No O3FA & O6FA Data)
0.017	Coffee, brewed from grounds w/ tap water, no sugar or cream (No O3FA Data)
0.010	Vegetable shortening, household, composite
0.010	Olive oil (Missing Trans Fat Data)

0.010	Water, bottled, Poland Spring
0.010	Sugars, granulated (sucrose)

Iron

Iron, mg/SS	Food
1.240	Thyme, dried
0.978	Parsley, dried (Missing O3FA Data)
0.827	Marjoram, dried
0.664	Cumin seed
0.642	Avg. Herbs
0.488	Dill weed, dried (Missing Data)
0.449	Celery seed
0.440	Oregano, dried
0.430	Bay leaf (Missing Data)
0.425	Cilantro, dried (No O3FA Data)
0.420	Basil, dried
0.414	Turmeric, ground
0.370	Anise seed (Missing Sugar, Vitamin, O3FA data)
0.344	Rice Krispies, Kellogg's
0.335	Fenugreek seed (Missing Vitamin & O3, 6FA Data)
0.323	Tarragon, dried (Missing Data)
0.318	Cheerios, General Mills
0.296	Curry powder
0.292	Rosemary, dried (Missing Data)
0.290	Corn Flakes, Kellogg's
0.289	Black pepper
0.281	Sage, ground
0.280	Wheaties, General Mills
0.280	Clams, mixed species, cooked in moist heat
0.270	Bran Flakes, single brand
0.266	Avg. Spice
0.261	Post Honey Bunches of Oats w/ Almonds (Missing Data)
0.236	Paprika
0.234	Frosted Flakes, Kellogg's
0.222	Cocoa Krispies, Kellogg's (No O3FA Data)
0.193	Cap'n Crunch with Crunch Berries, Quaker
0.192	Cap'n Crunch, Quaker
0.186	Apple Jacks, Kellogg's

0.185	Fennel seed (Missing Vitamin & O3FA Data)
0.184	Lucky Charms, General Mills
0.184	Peanut Butter Cap'n Crunch, Quaker
0.183	Cinnamon Toast Crunch cereal, ready-to-eat, General Mills
0.174	Thyme, fresh (Missing Data)
0.163	Coriander seed (Missing Data)
0.162	Caraway seed
0.150	Cocoa Puffs, General Mills
0.143	Chili powder
0.141	Froot Loops, General Mills
0.140	Cardamom (Missing Data)
0.139	Mace, ground (Missing Data)
0.128	Kellogg's Raisin Bran
0.120	Oysters, eastern, wild, cooked, moist heat
0.119	Spearmint, fresh (Missing Data)
0.111	Saffron (Missing Data)
0.100	Mustard seed, yellow
0.098	Poppy seed
0.093	Honeycomb cereal, Post, Kraft (low data)
0.087	Cloves, ground
0.083	Cinnamon
0.071	Allspice (Missing Data)
0.067	Golden Crisp, Post, Kraft
0.067	Oysters, eastern, wild, raw
0.066	Rosemarry, fresh (Missing Data)
0.063	Dark chocolate candies, 60-69% cacao solids (Missing Vitamin Data)
0.062	Corn Pops, Kellogg's
0.060	Cashews, dry roasted, no salt
0.057	Flaxseed
0.052	Pretzels, hard, plain, salted
0.051	Soybeans green, boiled, drained, no salt
0.050	Cream of Wheat, instant, prepared with water and salt
0.049	Kellogg's Nutri-Grain Cereal Bars, fruit-filled
0.047	Oats
0.046	White flour, white, all-purpose, enriched, bleached
0.046	Anchovies, European, canned in oil, drained solids

0.045	Ritz Crackers, Nabisco (Missing Vitamin Data)
0.044	Puffed Wheat, Quaker
0.044	Chocolate-flavored hazelnut spread (No Trans Fat Data)
0.042	Pistachio nuts, dry roasted, no salt
0.040	Soybeans (aka soy nuts) mature, dry roasted (Missing Sugar and Vitamin Data)
0.039	Whole wheat flour
0.039	Pretzels, soft
0.039	Ramen noodle soup, chicken flavor, dry
0.038	Sunflower Seeds, hulled, dry roasted, no salt
0.037	Almonds, USDA A256, A264
0.037	White bread, commercially prepared (inlcudes soft crumbs)
0.037	Kraft macaroni & cheese dinner, original, unprepared (Missing Data)
0.036	Wheat dinner rolls
0.036	Cake, snack cakes, crème-filled, chocolate with frosting
0.036	Barley (hulled)
0.036	Spinach, boiled, drained, no salt
0.035	Avg. Seafood
0.034	Avg. Nuts
0.034	Beef sticks, smoked (No Trans Fat Data)
0.033	Lentils, mature seeds, boiled, no salt
0.033	Roll, hard, kaiser
0.033	Pumpkin/Squash Seeds, dry roasted, no salt (Missing Vitamin & Se Data)
0.032	Matzo crackers, plain
0.032	Popcorn, air-popped
0.032	Ginger, ground
0.032	Basil, fresh
0.031	Whole wheat bread, prepared from recipe
0.031	Whole wheat pita bread
0.031	Shrimp, mixed species, cooked in moist heat
0.030	Scallops (bay & sea), steamed
0.030	Nutmeg, ground (Missing O3FA Data)
0.029	Kidney beans, red, boiled, no salt, mature seeds
0.029	Walnuts, USDA A259, A257
0.029	Popcorn, microwave, 94% fat free
0.029	Chick peas (garbanzo, bengal gram), mature seeds, boiled, no salt

0.028	T-bone steak, short loin, beef trimmed to 1/8" fat, all grades, broiled
0.028	Pecans, dry roasted, no salt
0.027	Pretzels, hard, whole-wheat (Missing Sugar Data)
0.027	Rye
0.027	Macadamia nuts, dry roasted, with salt
0.027	Macadamia nuts, dry roasted, w/out salt
0.026	White pita bread, enriched
0.026	Instant Oatmeal, Quaker, apples & cinnamon prepared w/ boiling water
0.025	Hamburger patty, 80/20 ground chuck beef, broiled
0.025	Lima beans, immature, boiled, drained, no salt
0.024	Coconut meat, raw
0.024	Avg. Beans & Lentils
0.024	Brazil nuts, dried, unblanched
0.024	Whole wheat bread, commecially prepared
0.024	Beef, eye of round, separable lean only, trimmed to 0" fat, all grades, roasted [cube steak]
0.024	Popcorn, regular butter flavor, microwave, made w/ partially hydrogenated oil (Missing Fats Data)
0.023	Milk chocolate candies (No Trans Fat Data)
0.023	Tortilla chips, plain, white corn
0.023	Swiss chard, boiled, drained, no salt
0.023	Peanuts, dry roasted, no salt, all types
0.023	Edamame beans, frozen, prepared
0.022	Granola bar, soft, uncoated, chocolate chip
0.022	Salami, cooked, beef (No Trans Fat Data)
0.022	Pastrami luncheon meat, beef, cured (No Trans Fat Data)
0.022	Salsa, USDA Commodity (Missing Sugar and Vitamin Data)
0.022	Peanut butter, smooth, USDA Commodity
0.022	Asparagus, raw
0.021	Slice of pizza, fast food, pizza chain, 14", cheese topping, regular crust (No Trans Fat Data)
0.021	Pinto beans, boiled, no salt, mature
0.021	Corned beef luncheon meat, beef, cured, canned (No Trans Fat Data)
0.021	Bologna, lebanon, beef (No O3FA Data)
0.020	Soy sauce, low sodium (soy & wheat)
0.020	Cheetos Crunchy cheese-flavored snacks (No O3, 6FA Data)
0.019	Soy sauce (soy & wheat)

0.019	Black beans, mature seeds, canned
0.019	Ground turkey, cooked
0.019	Raisins, seedless
0.018	Beets, canned, drained solids
0.018	Parboiled rice, white, long-grain, enriched, cooked
0.018	Cheese-flavor puffs or twists, corn-based
0.018	White rice, long-grain, pre-cooked or instant, prepared (Missing O3FA Data)
0.017	Mushrooms, boiled, drained, no salt
0.017	Teriyaki sauce, ready-to-serve
0.017	FritoLay Sun Chips, Multi-grain snack, original flavor
0.017	Popcorn, caramel-coated without peanuts
0.017	Garlic, raw
0.017	Avg. Cased Meat
0.016	Potato chips, plain, salted
0.016	Pepperoni, pork, beef
0.016	Tortilla chips, plain, yellow corn (Missing Vitamin Data)
0.015	Hummus, home prepared
0.015	Avg. Lean Meat
0.015	Mustard, prepared, yellow
0.015	Tuna fish, light, canned in water without salt, drained solids
0.015	Quinoa, cooked
0.015	Peas, frozen, boiled, drained, no salt
0.015	Egg noodles, cooked, enriched
0.015	Rice cakes, brown rice, plain
0.015	Turkey, fryer-roaster, breast meat only, roasted
0.014	Bacon (pork), cured, cooked, pan-fried
0.014	Sausage, Italian, pork, cooked (No Trans Fat Data)
0.014	Avg. Leafy Green Vegetables
0.014	Potato flour
0.014	Bagel, plain, unenriched w/ calcium propionate, onion, poppy, sesame (no cream cheese)
0.013	Chick peas (garbanzo, bengal gram), mature seeds, canned
0.013	Salami, dry or hard, pork (No Trans Fat Data)
0.013	Corn chips, extruded, plain
0.013	Banana chips
0.013	Honey Smacks, Kellogg's

0.013	Bologna, chicken, pork, beef
0.013	Hotdog, Oscar Mayer Wiener, beef frank (No Trans Fat Data)
0.013	Spaghetti, cooked, enriched w/out added salt, no sauce
0.012	Syrups, maple
0.012	White rice, long-grain, regular, cooked
0.012	Egg, whole, cooked, scrambled
0.012	Pork tenderloin lean, roasted, URMIS 3358
0.011	Crayfish, mixed species, farmed, cooked in moist heat
0.011	Chicken, broilers or fryers, breast, meat only (no skin), roasted
0.011	Potato, baked, flesh & skin, no salt
0.011	Potato, Russet, baked, flesh & skin
0.011	Pak-choi, boiled, drained, no salt
0.010	Salmon, Atlantic, wild, cooked in dry heat
0.010	Swordfish, cooked in dry heat
0.010	Tomato sauce, canned
0.010	Romaine or cos lettuce
0.010	Tuna fish, white, canned in water without salt, drained solids
0.009	Kale, boiled, drained, no salt
0.009	Pork-skins, plain
0.009	Parmesan cheese, grated (No Trans Fat Data)
0.009	Spam, Hormel (Missing Data)
0.009	Oats, unenriched, boiled, w/out salt
0.009	McDonald's French Fries
0.008	Beets, raw
0.008	Turkey, stuffing, mashed potatoes w/ gravy, assorted vegetables, frozen, microwaved
0.008	Mushrooms, canned, drained solids
0.007	Brown sugars
0.007	Banquest Hearty Ones Salisbury Steak Dinner w/ Gravy, Mashed Potatoes and Corn in Seasoned Sauce, frozen meal(Missing Data)
0.007	Candy bar, Snickers (King Size)
0.007	Potato, red, baked, flesh & skin
0.007	Sweet potato, baked in skin, no salt
0.007	Sesame sticks, wheat-based, salted
0.007	Tilapia, cooked in dry heat
0.007	Cheddar cheese (No Trans Fat Data)
0.007	Broccoli, boiled, drained, no salt

0.007	Raspberries, raw
0.006	Chicken noodle soup prepared with equal volume water
0.006	Snap (green string) beans, boiled, drained, no salt
0.006	Millet, cooked
0.006	Grits, corn, white, regular, quick, enriched, cooked with water, with salt
0.006	Wild rice, cooked
0.006	Mushrooms, portabella, raw
0.006	Butternut squash, winter, baked w/out salt, sugar or butter
0.006	Olive oil (Missing Trans Fat Data)
0.005	Avocado, raw, commercial varieties
0.005	Provolone cheese (No Trans Fat Data)
0.005	Avg. Vegetables
0.005	Banquet chicken pot pie, frozen entrée (Missing Data)
0.005	Olives, pickled, canned or bottled, green
0.005	Apricot jam and preserves
0.005	Hot Sauce (ready-to-serve, sauce, pepper or hot)
0.005	Ketchup
0.005	Avg. Cheese
0.005	Corn starch (Missing O3FA Data)
0.004	New England clam chowder, Campbell's Select (Missing Data)
0.004	Mozzarella cheese, whole milk (No Trans Fat Data)
0.004	Corn, sweet, yellow, boiled, drained, no salt
0.004	Mushrooms, shiitake, cooked, no salt
0.004	Lobster, northern, cooked in moist heat
0.004	Honey
0.004	Brown rice, long-grain, cooked
0.004	Peppers, sweet, red, raw
0.004	Cauliflower, raw
0.004	Iceberg lettuce
0.004	Horseradish, prepared
0.004	McDonald's spicy buffalo sauce
0.004	McDonald's barbeque sauce
0.004	Ricotta cheese, whole milk (No Trans Fat Data)
0.004	American cheese, pasteurized, w/out disodium phosphate (No Trans Fat Data)
0.004	Whiting, mixed species, cooked in dry heat

0.004	Strawberries, raw
0.004	Cream cheese (No Trans Fat Data)
0.004	Pickles, cucumber, dill or kosher dill
0.004	Cherries, sweet, raw
0.003	Radishes, raw
0.003	Salt (table salt)
0.003	Peppers, sweet, green, raw
0.003	Zucchini, summer squash, w/ skin, boiled w/out salt, drained
0.003	Grapes, red or green, European type such as Thompson seedless, raw
0.003	Spaghetti squash, winter, boiled w/out salt, drained
0.003	Flounder (sole), cooked in dry heat
0.003	Weight Watchers Smart Ones Chicken Enchiladas Suiza, Sour Cream w/ Cheese frozen entrée (Missing Data)
0.003	Carrots, raw, USDA A099
0.003	Pineapple, raw, all varieties
0.003	Pomegranate, raw
0.003	Blueberries, raw
0.003	Eggplant, boiled, drained, no salt
0.003	Light mayo (salad dressing)
0.003	Blue Cheese (No Trans Fat Data)
0.003	Banana, raw
0.003	Pineapple, canned, juice pack, drained
0.003	Avg. Fruit
0.003	Tomatoes, raw, red, ripe
0.003	Cucumber, raw w/ peel
0.002	Mashed potatoes, home-prepared, whole milk & butter added
0.002	Grape Juice, canned or bottled, unsweetened
0.002	Red snapper, cooked, dry heat
0.002	Peaches, raw
0.002	Mayonnaise, soybean oil, w/ salt (salad dressing)
0.002	Swiss Cheese (No Trans Fat Data)
0.002	Cabbage, boiled, drained, no salt
0.002	Ice cream, soft-serve, french vanilla (No Trans Fat Data)
0.002	Mozzarella cheese, part skim (No Trans Fat Data)
0.002	Velveeta cheese, Kraft, pasteurized spread (Missing Data)
0.002	Acerola (West Indian cherry), raw (Missing Sugar and Vitamin Data)

0.002	Cantaloupe, raw
0.002	Onion, raw
0.002	Ginger Ale
0.001	Apple, raw, with skin A343
0.001	Cottage cheese, 1% milkfat (No Trans Fat Data)
0.001	Swanson chicken broth, 99% Fat Free
0.001	Mangos, raw
0.001	Cranberry juice cocktail, bottled
0.001	Sprite
0.001	White rice, glutinous, cooked
0.001	Apple Juice, canned or bottled, unsweetened
0.001	Rice noodles, cooked (Missing Sugar & Unsaturated Fat Data)
0.001	Orange, raw, all commercial varieties
0.001	Ice creams, vanilla (No Trans Fat Data)
0.001	Margarine (vegetable oil spread, 70% fat, soybean & partially hydrogenated soybean, stick)
0.001	Chamomile Tea (No O3FA & O6FA Data)
0.001	Yogurt, regular low-fat, plain, 12 g protein per 8 oz
0.001	Papayas, raw

Magnesium

Magnesium, mg/SS	Food
6.940	Cilantro, dried (No O3FA Data)
4.510	Dill weed, dried (Missing Data)
4.490	Celery seed
4.280	Sage, ground
4.220	Basil, dried
3.920	Flaxseed
3.850	Fennel seed (Missing Vitamin & O3FA Data)
3.759	Brazil nuts, dried, unblanched
3.660	Cumin seed
3.470	Poppy seed
3.470	Tarragon, dried (Missing Data)
3.460	Marjoram, dried
3.372	Avg. Herbs
3.300	Coriander seed (Missing Data)
2.980	Mustard seed, yellow
2.700	Oregano, dried
2.678	Almonds, USDA A256, A264
2.640	Cloves, ground
2.640	Saffron (Missing Data)
2.620	Pumpkin/Squash Seeds, dry roasted, no salt (Missing Vitamin & Se Data)
2.599	Cashews, dry roasted, no salt
2.580	Caraway seed
2.540	Curry powder
2.490	Parsley, dried (Missing O3FA Data)
2.446	Avg. Spice
2.290	Cardamom (Missing Data)
2.279	Soybeans (aka soy nuts) mature, dry roasted (Missing Sugar and Vitamin Data)
2.200	Thyme, dried
2.200	Rosemary, dried (Missing Data)
2.140	Bran Flakes, single brand
1.940	Black pepper
1.930	Turmeric, ground

1.910	Fenugreek seed (Missing Vitamin & O3, 6FA Data)
1.850	Paprika
1.830	Nutmeg, ground (Missing O3FA Data)
1.791	Peanut butter, smooth, USDA Commodity
1.769	Oats
1.760	Peanuts, dry roasted, no salt, all types
1.759	Dark chocolate candies, 60-69% cacao solids (Missing Vitamin Data)
1.700	Chili powder
1.700	Anise seed (Missing Sugar, Vitamin, O3FA data)
1.644	Avg. Nuts
1.630	Mace, ground (Missing Data)
1.600	Thyme, fresh (Missing Data)
1.581	Walnuts, USDA A259, A257
1.460	Tortilla chips, plain, white corn
1.440	Popcorn, air-popped
1.383	Whole wheat flour
1.350	Allspice (Missing Data)
1.332	Barley (hulled)
1.330	Puffed Wheat, Quaker
1.320	Pecans, dry roasted, no salt
1.310	Rice cakes, brown rice, plain
1.289	Sunflower Seeds, hulled, dry roased, no salt
1.260	Kellogg's Raisin Bran
1.240	Popcorn, microwave, 94% fat free
1.207	Rye
1.203	Pistachio nuts, dry roasted, no salt
1.200	Cheerios, General Mills
1.200	Bay leaf (Missing Data)
1.182	Macadamia nuts, dry roasted, with salt
1.182	Macadamia nuts, dry roasted, w/out salt
1.070	Wheaties, General Mills
0.950	Oysters, eastern, wild, cooked, moist heat
0.920	Popcorn, regular butter flavor, microwave, made w/ partially hydrogenated oil (Missing Fats Data)
0.910	Rosemarry, fresh (Missing Data)
0.872	Spinach, boiled, drained, no salt

0.870	Tortilla chips, plain, yellow corn (Missing Vitamin Data)
0.860	Soybeans green, boiled, drained, no salt
0.857	Swiss chard, boiled, drained, no salt
0.838	Corn chips, extruded, plain
0.820	Whole wheat bread, commecially prepared
0.810	Whole wheat bread, prepared from recipe
0.760	Banana chips
0.760	FritoLay Sun Chips, Multi-grain snack, original flavor
0.741	Lima beans, immature, boiled, drained, no salt
0.720	Candy bar, Snickers (King Size)
0.700	Potato chips, plain, salted
0.700	Peanut Butter Cap'n Crunch, Quaker
0.690	Whole wheat pita bread
0.690	Anchovies, European, canned in oil, drained solids
0.690	Post Honey Bunches of Oats w/ Almonds (Missing Data)
0.650	Potato flour
0.640	Edamame beans, frozen, prepared
0.640	Granola bar, soft, uncoated, chocolate chip
0.640	Chocolate-flavored hazelnut spread (No Trans Fat Data)
0.640	Basil, fresh
0.638	Quinoa, cooked
0.631	Milk chocolate candies (No Trans Fat Data)
0.630	Spearmint, fresh (Missing Data)
0.611	Teriyaki sauce, ready-to-serve
0.610	Golden Crisp, Post, Kraft
0.600	Cinnamon
0.590	Lucky Charms, General Mills
0.590	Honey Smacks, Kellogg's
0.580	Flounder (sole), cooked in dry heat
0.550	Scallops (bay & sea), steamed
0.540	Cap'n Crunch, Quaker
0.540	Cap'n Crunch with Crunch Berries, Quaker
0.515	Ginger, ground
0.500	Pinto beans, boiled, no salt, mature
0.490	Mustard, prepared, yellow
0.480	Chick peas (garbanzo, bengal gram), mature seeds, boiled, no

	salt
0.472	Oysters, eastern, wild, raw
0.461	Avg. Beans & Lentils
0.450	Sesame sticks, wheat-based, salted
0.450	Kidney beans, red, boiled, no salt, mature seeds
0.440	Millet, cooked
0.431	Soy sauce (soy & wheat)
0.430	Brown rice, long-grain, cooked
0.420	Cinnamon Toast Crunch cereal, ready-to-eat, General Mills
0.388	Avg. Seafood
0.380	Swiss Cheese (No Trans Fat Data)
0.380	Parmesan cheese, grated (No Trans Fat Data)
0.380	Cocoa Krispies, Kellogg's (No O3FA Data)
0.370	Salmon, Atlantic, wild, cooked in dry heat
0.370	Red snapper, cooked, dry heat
0.370	Honeycomb cereal, Post, Kraft (low data)
0.360	Lentils, mature seeds, boiled, no salt
0.360	Wheat dinner rolls
0.360	Cake, snack cakes, crème-filled, chocolate with frosting
0.360	Bacon (pork), cured, cooked, pan-fried
0.360	Avg. Leafy Green Vegetables
0.350	Lobster, northern, cooked in moist heat
0.350	Black beans, mature seeds, canned
0.350	Popcorn, caramel-coated without peanuts
0.340	Soy sauce, low sodium (soy & wheat)
0.340	Shrimp, mixed species, cooked in moist heat
0.340	Tilapia, cooked in dry heat
0.340	Swordfish, cooked in dry heat
0.330	Tuna fish, white, canned in water without salt, drained solids
0.330	Crayfish, mixed species, farmed, cooked in moist heat
0.320	Wild rice, cooked
0.320	Raisins, seedless
0.320	Coconut meat, raw
0.320	McDonald's French Fries
0.300	Potato, Russet, baked, flesh & skin
0.300	Pretzels, hard, whole-wheat (Missing Sugar Data)

0.290	Bagel, plain, unenriched w/ calcium propionate, onion, poppy, sesame (no cream cheese)
0.290	Avocado, raw, commercial varieties
0.290	Chicken, broilers or fryers, breast, meat only (no skin), roasted
0.290	Chick peas (garbanzo, bengal gram), mature seeds, canned
0.290	Pretzels, hard, plain, salted
0.290	Turkey, fryer-roaster, breast meat only, roasted
0.290	Pork tenderloin lean, roasted, URMIS 3358
0.290	Hummus, home prepared
0.290	Butternut squash, winter, baked w/out salt, sugar or butter
0.280	Cheddar cheese (No Trans Fat Data)
0.280	Provolone cheese (No Trans Fat Data)
0.280	Potato, baked, flesh & skin, no salt
0.280	Potato, red, baked, flesh & skin
0.270	Tuna fish, light, canned in water without salt, drained solids
0.270	Oats, unenriched, boiled, w/out salt
0.270	Sweet potato, baked in skin, no salt
0.270	Roll, hard, kaiser
0.270	Kellogg's Nutri-Grain Cereal Bars, fruit-filled
0.270	Horseradish, prepared
0.270	Cocoa Puffs, General Mills
0.270	Whiting, mixed species, cooked in dry heat
0.270	Banana, raw
0.265	Avg. Lean Meat
0.260	White pita bread, enriched
0.260	Rice Krispies, Kellogg's
0.260	Corn, sweet, yellow, boiled, drained, no salt
0.250	Garlic, raw
0.250	Matzo crackers, plain
0.241	Avg. Cheese
0.240	T-bone steak, short loin, beef trimmed to 1/8" fat, all grades, broiled
0.240	Ground turkey, cooked
0.240	Slice of pizza, fast food, pizza chain, 14", cheese topping, regular crust (No Trans Fat Data)
0.230	Beets, raw
0.230	White bread, commercially prepared (inlcudes soft crumbs)

0.230	Froot Loops, General Mills
0.230	Blue Cheese (No Trans Fat Data)
0.230	Mozzarella cheese, part skim (No Trans Fat Data)
0.220	Salami, dry or hard, pork (No Trans Fat Data)
0.220	Raspberries, raw
0.220	Peas, frozen, boiled, drained, no salt
0.220	Zucchini, summer squash, w/ skin, boiled w/out salt, drained
0.220	White flour, white, all-purpose, enriched, bleached
0.220	American cheese, pasteurized, w/out disodium phosphate (No Trans Fat Data)
0.220	Ramen noodle soup, chicken flavor, dry
0.210	Egg noodles, cooked, enriched
0.210	Broccoli, boiled, drained, no salt
0.210	Apple Jacks, Kellogg's
0.210	Pepperoni, pork, beef
0.210	Beef sticks, smoked (No Trans Fat Data)
0.210	Pretzels, soft
0.200	Hamburger patty, 80/20 ground chuck beef, broiled
0.200	Bologna, lebanon, beef (No O3FA Data)
0.200	Mozzarella cheese, whole milk (No Trans Fat Data)
0.190	Cheese-flavor puffs or twists, corn-based
0.190	Ritz Crackers, Nabisco (Missing Vitamin Data)
0.190	Ketchup
0.190	Beef, eye of round, separable lean only, trimmed to 0" fat, all grades, roasted [cube steak]
0.190	Instant Oatmeal, Quaker, apples & cinnamon prepared w/ boiling water
0.180	Kale, boiled, drained, no salt
0.180	Snap (green string) beans, boiled, drained, no salt
0.180	Spaghetti, cooked, enriched w/out added salt, no sauce
0.180	Clams, mixed species, cooked in moist heat
0.180	Sausage, Italian, pork, cooked (No Trans Fat Data)
0.180	Mashed potatoes, home-prepared, whole milk & butter added
0.180	Acerola (West Indian cherry), raw (Missing Sugar and Vitamin Data)
0.180	Turkey, stuffing, mashed potatoes w/ gravy, assorted vegetables, frozen, microwaved
0.170	Yogurt, regular low-fat, plain, 12 g protein per 8 oz

0.170	Beets, canned, drained solids
0.170	Pastrami luncheon meat, beef, cured (No Trans Fat Data)
0.166	Avg. Cased Meat
0.160	Tomato sauce, canned
0.160	Salsa, USDA Commodity (Missing Sugar and Vitamin Data)
0.150	Cauliflower, raw
0.150	Cabbage, boiled, drained, no salt
0.150	Bologna, chicken, pork, beef
0.150	Mushrooms, canned, drained solids
0.150	Pineapple, canned, juice pack, drained
0.147	Avg. Vegetables
0.140	Asparagus, raw
0.140	Syrups, maple
0.140	Mushrooms, shiitake, cooked, no salt
0.140	Romaine or cos lettuce
0.140	Ice creams, vanilla (No Trans Fat Data)
0.140	Corned beef luncheon meat, beef, cured, canned (No Trans Fat Data)
0.140	Spam, Hormel (Missing Data)
0.130	Strawberries, raw
0.130	McDonald's barbeque sauce
0.130	Salami, cooked, beef (No Trans Fat Data)
0.130	Hotdog, Oscar Mayer Wiener, beef frank (No Trans Fat Data)
0.130	Cucumber, raw w/ peel
0.120	Carrots, raw, USDA A099
0.120	White rice, long-grain, regular, cooked
0.120	Peppers, sweet, red, raw
0.120	Pineapple, raw, all varieties
0.120	Pomegranate, raw
0.120	Ice cream, soft-serve, french vanilla (No Trans Fat Data)
0.120	Egg, whole, cooked, scrambled
0.120	Mushrooms, boiled, drained, no salt
0.120	Cantaloupe, raw
0.118	Avg. Fruit
0.110	Spaghetti squash, winter, boiled w/out salt, drained
0.110	Milk, nonfat, added Vit A

0.110	Cherries, sweet, raw
0.110	Milk, nonfat, Ca fortified
0.110	Tomatoes, raw, red, ripe
0.110	Mushrooms, portabella, raw
0.110	Eggplant, boiled, drained, no salt
0.110	Pak-choi, boiled, drained, no salt
0.110	Olives, pickled, canned or bottled, green
0.110	Pork-skins, plain
0.110	Ricotta cheese, whole milk (No Trans Fat Data)
0.110	Milk, lowfat, 1%, added Vit A
0.110	Milk, reduced fat, 2%, added Vit A
0.102	Orange, raw, all commercial varieties
0.100	Papayas, raw
0.100	Peppers, sweet, green, raw
0.100	Onion, raw
0.100	Grape Juice, canned or bottled, unsweetened
0.100	Radishes, raw
0.100	Milk, whole, 3.25% milkfat
0.090	Cream cheese (No Trans Fat Data)
0.090	Brown sugars
0.090	Corn Flakes, Kellogg's
0.090	Parboiled rice, white, long-grain, enriched, cooked
0.090	Peaches, raw
0.090	Mangos, raw
0.070	Pickles, cucumber, dill or kosher dill
0.070	Grapes, red or green, European type such as Thompson seedless, raw
0.070	Iceberg lettuce
0.070	Corn Pops, Kellogg's
0.070	Frosted Flakes, Kellogg's
0.060	Cream of Wheat, instant, prepared with water and salt
0.060	Blueberries, raw
0.060	McDonald's spicy buffalo sauce
0.060	Margarine, industrial, non-dairy, cottonseed, soy oil (partially hydrogenated), for flaky pastries
0.060	Lemon juice, raw
0.050	White rice, long-grain, pre-cooked or instant, prepared (Missing

	O3FA Data)
0.050	Apple, raw, with skin A343
0.050	Hot Sauce (ready-to-serve, sauce, pepper or hot)
0.050	Cottage cheese, 1% milkfat (No Trans Fat Data)
0.050	White rice, glutinous, cooked
0.050	Apple Juice, canned or bottled, unsweetened
0.050	Grits, corn, white, regular, quick, enriched, cooked with water, with salt
0.040	Apricot jam and preserves
0.040	Chicken noodle soup prepared with equal volume water
0.030	Rice noodles, cooked (Missing Sugar & Unsaturated Fat Data)
0.030	Black Tea, brewed with tap water
0.030	Corn starch (Missing O3FA Data)
0.026	Coffee, brewed from grounds w/ tap water, no sugar or cream (No O3FA Data)
0.020	Honey
0.020	Light mayo (salad dressing)
0.020	Margarine (vegetable oil spread, 70% fat, soybean & partially hydrogenated soybean, stick)
0.020	Butter, salted (No Trans Fat Data)
0.010	Swanson chicken broth, 99% Fat Free
0.010	Chamomile Tea (No O3FA & O6FA Data)
0.010	Water, tap, drinking
0.010	Water, bottled, Poland Spring
0.010	Sprite
0.010	Ginger Ale
0.010	Mayonnaise, soybean oil, w/ salt (salad dressing)
0.010	Salt (table salt)
0.010	Cranberry juice cocktail, bottled

Phosphorus

Phosphorus, mg/SS	Food
11.547	Sunflower Seeds, hulled, dry roased, no salt
9.480	Chia seeds, dried (Missing Sugar and Vitamin Data)
8.700	Poppy seed
8.630	Velveeta cheese, Kraft, pasteurized spread (Missing Data)
8.410	Mustard seed, yellow
7.290	Parmesan cheese, grated (No Trans Fat Data)
7.248	Brazil nuts, dried, unblanched
6.488	Soybeans (aka soy nuts) mature, dry roasted (Missing Sugar and Vitamin Data)
6.420	Flaxseed
5.680	Caraway seed
5.667	Swiss Cheese (No Trans Fat Data)
5.610	Bacon (pork), cured, cooked, pan-fried
5.470	Celery seed
5.430	Dill weed, dried (Missing Data)
5.231	Oats
5.121	Cheddar cheese (No Trans Fat Data)
5.080	Bran Flakes, single brand
4.990	Cumin seed
4.962	Provolone cheese (No Trans Fat Data)
4.900	Basil, dried
4.898	Cashews, dry roasted, no salt
4.870	Fennel seed (Missing Vitamin & O3FA Data)
4.854	Pistachio nuts, dry roasted, no salt
4.839	Almonds, USDA A256, A264
4.810	Cilantro, dried (No O3FA Data)
4.630	Mozzarella cheese, part skim (No Trans Fat Data)
4.452	Avg. Nuts
4.440	American cheese, pasteurized, w/out disodium phosphate (No Trans Fat Data)
4.400	Anise seed (Missing Sugar, Vitamin, O3FA data)
4.350	Cheerios, General Mills
4.170	Avg. Cheese
4.090	Coriander seed (Missing Data)

3.870	Blue Cheese (No Trans Fat Data)
3.780	Kraft macaroni & cheese dinner, original, unprepared (Missing Data)
3.740	Rye
3.693	Avg. Spice
3.650	Kellogg's Raisin Bran
3.600	Rice cakes, brown rice, plain
3.582	Peanuts, dry roasted, no salt, all types
3.580	Popcorn, air-popped
3.536	Mozzarella cheese, whole milk (No Trans Fat Data)
3.510	Parsley, dried (Missing O3FA Data)
3.490	Curry powder
3.462	Walnuts, USDA A259, A257
3.458	Whole wheat flour
3.450	Paprika
3.380	Scallops (bay & sea), steamed
3.380	Clams, mixed species, cooked in moist heat
3.368	Swordfish, cooked in dry heat
3.349	Peanut butter, smooth, USDA Commodity
3.330	Wheaties, General Mills
3.310	Puffed Wheat, Quaker
3.130	Tarragon, dried (Missing Data)
3.060	Marjoram, dried
3.040	Popcorn, microwave, 94% fat free
3.030	Chili powder
2.960	Fenugreek seed (Missing Vitamin & O3, 6FA Data)
2.930	Pecans, dry roasted, no salt
2.890	Flounder (sole), cooked in dry heat
2.850	Whiting, mixed species, cooked in dry heat
2.730	Ritz Crackers, Nabisco (Missing Vitamin Data)
2.680	Turmeric, ground
2.670	Pork tenderloin lean, roasted, URMIS 3358
2.641	Barley (hulled)
2.598	Dark chocolate candies, 60-69% cacao solids (Missing Vitamin Data)
2.576	Avg. Herbs
2.558	Salmon, Atlantic, wild, cooked in dry heat

2.520	Anchovies, European, canned in oil, drained solids
2.520	Saffron (Missing Data)
2.448	Soybeans green, boiled, drained, no salt
2.429	Avg. Seafood
2.410	Crayfish, mixed species, farmed, cooked in moist heat
2.370	Lucky Charms, General Mills
2.360	Tortilla chips, plain, yellow corn (Missing Vitamin Data)
2.340	Popcorn, regular butter flavor, microwave, made w/ partially hydrogenated oil (Missing Fats Data)
2.292	Salami, dry or hard, pork (No Trans Fat Data)
2.279	Chicken, broilers or fryers, breast, meat only (no skin), roasted
2.270	Bologna, chicken, pork, beef
2.257	Avg. Lean Meat
2.240	Turkey, fryer-roaster, breast meat only, roasted
2.220	FritoLay Sun Chips, Multi-grain snack, original flavor
2.169	Tuna fish, white, canned in water without salt, drained solids
2.130	Nutmeg, ground (Missing O3FA Data)
2.117	Slice of pizza, fast food, pizza chain, 14", cheese topping, regular crust (No Trans Fat Data)
2.077	Milk chocolate candies (No Trans Fat Data)
2.050	Salami, cooked, beef (No Trans Fat Data)
2.040	Tilapia, cooked in dry heat
2.030	Oysters, eastern, wild, cooked, moist heat
2.020	Whole wheat bread, commecially prepared
2.012	Red snapper, cooked, dry heat
2.010	Thyme, dried
2.000	Tortilla chips, plain, white corn
2.000	Oregano, dried
1.977	Macadamia nuts, dry roasted, with salt
1.977	Macadamia nuts, dry roasted, w/out salt
1.960	Ground turkey, cooked
1.950	Peanut Butter Cap'n Crunch, Quaker
1.940	Hamburger patty, 80/20 ground chuck beef, broiled
1.930	T-bone steak, short loin, beef trimmed to 1/8" fat, all grades, broiled
1.920	Post Honey Bunches of Oats w/ Almonds (Missing Data)
1.920	Bologna, lebanon, beef (No O3FA Data)

1.903	Candy bar, Snickers (King Size)
1.870	Whole wheat bread, prepared from recipe
1.848	Lobster, northern, cooked in moist heat
1.840	Beef, eye of round, separable lean only, trimmed to 0" fat, all grades, roasted [cube steak]
1.800	Whole wheat pita bread
1.800	Beef sticks, smoked (No Trans Fat Data)
1.798	Lentils, mature seeds, boiled, no salt
1.793	Avg. Cased Meat
1.780	Cardamom (Missing Data)
1.770	Pepperoni, pork, beef
1.760	Granola bar, soft, uncoated, chocolate chip
1.750	Pastrami luncheon meat, beef, cured (No Trans Fat Data)
1.730	Black pepper
1.710	Honey Smacks, Kellogg's
1.700	Egg, whole, cooked, scrambled
1.700	Sausage, Italian, pork, cooked (No Trans Fat Data)
1.690	Edamame beans, frozen, prepared
1.683	Chick peas (garbanzo, bengal gram), mature seeds, boiled, no salt
1.681	Potato flour
1.660	Cap'n Crunch, Quaker
1.660	Cap'n Crunch with Crunch Berries, Quaker
1.630	Tuna fish, light, canned in water without salt, drained solids
1.600	Cinnamon Toast Crunch cereal, ready-to-eat, General Mills
1.580	Ricotta cheese, whole milk (No Trans Fat Data)
1.571	Corn chips, extruded, plain
1.551	Potato chips, plain, salted
1.542	Teriyaki sauce, ready-to-serve
1.529	Garlic, raw
1.520	Chocolate-flavored hazelnut spread (No Trans Fat Data)
1.519	Quinoa, cooked
1.468	Pinto beans, boiled, no salt, mature
1.441	Yogurt, regular low-fat, plain, 12 g protein per 8 oz
1.418	Kidney beans, red, boiled, no salt, mature seeds
1.400	Hotdog, Oscar Mayer Wiener, beef frank (No Trans Fat Data)
1.380	Sesame sticks, wheat-based, salted

1.370	Shrimp, mixed species, cooked in moist heat
1.360	Golden Crisp, Post, Kraft
1.351	Oysters, eastern, wild, raw
1.349	Avg. Beans & Lentils
1.341	Cottage cheese, 1% milkfat (No Trans Fat Data)
1.316	McDonald's French Fries
1.300	Mushrooms, portabella, raw
1.300	Lima beans, immature, boiled, drained, no salt
1.280	Cheese-flavor puffs or twists, corn-based
1.260	Rice Krispies, Kellogg's
1.251	Soy sauce (soy & wheat)
1.250	Pretzels, hard, whole-wheat (Missing Sugar Data)
1.180	Ramen noodle soup, chicken flavor, dry
1.160	Ice cream, soft-serve, french vanilla (No Trans Fat Data)
1.131	Coconut meat, raw
1.130	Pretzels, hard, plain, salted
1.130	Allspice (Missing Data)
1.130	Bay leaf (Missing Data)
1.110	Corned beef luncheon meat, beef, cured, canned (No Trans Fat Data)
1.102	Hummus, home prepared
1.100	Mace, ground (Missing Data)
1.098	Soy sauce, low sodium (soy & wheat)
1.080	White flour, white, all-purpose, enriched, bleached
1.079	Black beans, mature seeds, canned
1.060	Cream cheese (No Trans Fat Data)
1.060	Mustard, prepared, yellow
1.060	Thyme, fresh (Missing Data)
1.060	Turkey, stuffing, mashed potatoes w/ gravy, assorted vegetables, frozen, microwaved
1.050	Ice creams, vanilla (No Trans Fat Data)
1.050	Cloves, ground
1.040	Wheat dinner rolls
1.030	Kellogg's Nutri-Grain Cereal Bars, fruit-filled
1.020	Cocoa Krispies, Kellogg's (No O3FA Data)
1.012	Raisins, seedless
1.008	Milk, nonfat, added Vit A

1.008	Milk, nonfat, Ca fortified
1.000	Millet, cooked
1.000	Roll, hard, kaiser
0.990	White bread, commercially prepared (inlcudes soft crumbs)
0.970	White pita bread, enriched
0.962	Bagel, plain, unenriched w/ calcium propionate, onion, poppy, sesame (no cream cheese)
0.951	Milk, lowfat, 1%, added Vit A
0.939	Milk, reduced fat, 2%, added Vit A
0.930	Honeycomb cereal, Post, Kraft (low data)
0.920	Pumpkin/Squash Seeds, dry roasted, no salt (Missing Vitamin & Se Data)
0.910	Sage, ground
0.910	Milk, whole, 3.25% milkfat
0.900	Chick peas (garbanzo, bengal gram), mature seeds, canned
0.890	Matzo crackers, plain
0.872	Mushrooms, boiled, drained, no salt
0.870	Cake, snack cakes, crème-filled, chocolate with frosting
0.850	Pork-skins, plain
0.831	Brown rice, long-grain, cooked
0.830	Popcorn, caramel-coated without peanuts
0.817	Wild rice, cooked
0.790	Pretzels, soft
0.780	Apple Jacks, Kellogg's
0.771	Peas, frozen, boiled, drained, no salt
0.769	Oats, unenriched, boiled, w/out salt
0.763	Egg noodles, cooked, enriched
0.750	Corn, sweet, yellow, boiled, drained, no salt
0.719	Potato, red, baked, flesh & skin
0.709	Potato, Russet, baked, flesh & skin
0.700	Rosemary, dried (Missing Data)
0.699	Potato, baked, flesh & skin, no salt
0.671	Broccoli, boiled, drained, no salt
0.670	Cocoa Puffs, General Mills
0.660	Mushrooms, canned, drained solids
0.660	Rosemarry, fresh (Missing Data)
0.640	Froot Loops, General Mills

0.640	Cinnamon
0.630	Instant Oatmeal, Quaker, apples & cinnamon prepared w/ boiling water
0.600	Spearmint, fresh (Missing Data)
0.580	Spaghetti, cooked, enriched w/out added salt, no sauce
0.561	Spinach, boiled, drained, no salt
0.560	Banana chips
0.560	Basil, fresh
0.550	Parboiled rice, white, long-grain, enriched, cooked
0.540	Sweet potato, baked in skin, no salt
0.522	Avocado, raw, commercial varieties
0.520	Asparagus, raw
0.510	Margarine, industrial, non-dairy, cottonseed, soy oil (partially hydrogenated), for flaky pastries
0.460	Mashed potatoes, home-prepared, whole milk & butter added
0.440	Cauliflower, raw
0.430	White rice, long-grain, regular, cooked
0.414	Ginger, ground
0.410	Frosted Flakes, Kellogg's
0.400	Zucchini, summer squash, w/ skin, boiled w/out salt, drained
0.400	Beets, raw
0.395	Avg. Leafy Green Vegetables
0.370	White rice, long-grain, pre-cooked or instant, prepared (Missing O3FA Data)
0.370	Corn Flakes, Kellogg's
0.360	Pomegranate, raw
0.350	Carrots, raw, USDA A099
0.350	Light mayo (salad dressing)
0.337	Avg. Vegetables
0.330	Swiss chard, boiled, drained, no salt
0.330	Cabbage, boiled, drained, no salt
0.330	Ketchup
0.310	Horseradish, prepared
0.310	Corn Pops, Kellogg's
0.300	Romaine or cos lettuce
0.300	McDonald's barbeque sauce
0.300	Salsa, USDA Commodity (Missing Sugar and Vitamin Data)

0.290	Raspberries, raw
0.290	Onion, raw
0.290	Pak-choi, boiled, drained, no salt
0.290	Mushrooms, shiitake, cooked, no salt
0.290	Snap (green string) beans, boiled, drained, no salt
0.280	Kale, boiled, drained, no salt
0.270	Butternut squash, winter, baked w/out salt, sugar or butter
0.260	Tomato sauce, canned
0.260	Peppers, sweet, red, raw
0.250	Mayonnaise, soybean oil, w/ salt (salad dressing)
0.240	Tomatoes, raw, red, ripe
0.240	Strawberries, raw
0.240	Butter, salted (No Trans Fat Data)
0.240	Cucumber, raw w/ peel
0.220	Banana, raw
0.210	Cherries, sweet, raw
0.200	Peaches, raw
0.200	Peppers, sweet, green, raw
0.200	Iceberg lettuce
0.200	Rice noodles, cooked (Missing Sugar & Unsaturated Fat Data)
0.200	Grapes, red or green, European type such as Thompson seedless, raw
0.200	Radishes, raw
0.180	Cream of Wheat, instant, prepared with water and salt
0.177	Avg. Fruit
0.170	Chicken noodle soup prepared with equal volume water
0.170	Beets, canned, drained solids
0.150	Cantaloupe, raw
0.150	Eggplant, boiled, drained, no salt
0.143	Orange, raw, all commercial varieties
0.140	Spaghetti squash, winter, boiled w/out salt, drained
0.140	Grape Juice, canned or bottled, unsweetened
0.130	Corn starch (Missing O3FA Data)
0.120	Pickles, cucumber, dill or kosher dill
0.120	Blueberries, raw
0.110	Mangos, raw

0.110	Swanson chicken broth, 99% Fat Free
0.110	Hot Sauce (ready-to-serve, sauce, pepper or hot)
0.110	McDonald's spicy buffalo sauce
0.110	Acerola (West Indian cherry), raw (Missing Sugar and Vitamin Data)
0.110	Grits, corn, white, regular, quick, enriched, cooked with water, with salt
0.110	Apple, raw, with skin A343
0.100	Margarine (vegetable oil spread, 70% fat, soybean & partially hydrogenated soybean, stick)
0.080	Pineapple, raw, all varieties
0.080	White rice, glutinous, cooked
0.070	Pineapple, canned, juice pack, drained
0.070	Apple Juice, canned or bottled, unsweetened
0.060	Lemon juice, raw
0.050	Papayas, raw
0.040	Honey
0.040	Olives, pickled, canned or bottled, green
0.040	Brown sugars
0.030	Apricot jam and preserves
0.026	Coffee, brewed from grounds w/ tap water, no sugar or cream (No O3FA Data)
0.020	Syrups, maple
0.010	Black Tea, brewed with tap water
0.010	Cranberry juice cocktail, bottled

Potassium

Potassium, mg/SS	Food
44.660	Cilantro, dried (No O3FA Data)
38.050	Parsley, dried (Missing O3FA Data)
34.330	Basil, dried
33.080	Dill weed, dried (Missing Data)
30.200	Tarragon, dried (Missing Data)
25.250	Turmeric, ground
23.440	Paprika
19.160	Chili powder
17.880	Cumin seed
17.240	Saffron (Missing Data)
17.016	Avg. Herbs
16.940	Fennel seed (Missing Vitamin & O3FA Data)
16.690	Oregano, dried
16.419	Potato chips, plain, salted
15.430	Curry powder
15.220	Marjoram, dried
14.855	Avg. Spice
14.410	Anise seed (Missing Sugar, Vitamin, O3FA data)
14.000	Celery seed
13.640	Soybeans (aka soy nuts) mature, dry roasted (Missing Sugar and Vitamin Data)
13.510	Caraway seed
12.670	Coriander seed (Missing Data)
12.590	Black pepper
11.190	Cardamom (Missing Data)
11.020	Cloves, ground
10.700	Sage, ground
10.440	Allspice (Missing Data)
10.423	Pistachio nuts, dry roasted, no salt
10.013	Potato flour
9.550	Rosemary, dried (Missing Data)
9.190	Pumpkin/Squash Seeds, dry roasted, no salt (Missing Vitamin & Se Data)
8.500	Sunflower Seeds, hulled, dry roased, no salt

8.140	Thyme, dried
8.130	Flaxseed
7.700	Fenugreek seed (Missing Vitamin & O3, 6FA Data)
7.491	Raisins, seedless
7.190	Poppy seed
7.049	Almonds, USDA A256, A264
7.000	Wheaties, General Mills
6.820	Mustard seed, yellow
6.680	Rosemarry, fresh (Missing Data)
6.586	Brazil nuts, dried, unblanched
6.582	Peanuts, dry roasted, no salt, all types
6.280	Clams, mixed species, cooked in moist heat
6.279	Salmon, Atlantic, wild, cooked in dry heat
6.160	Bran Flakes, single brand
6.090	Cheerios, General Mills
6.090	Thyme, fresh (Missing Data)
6.012	Avg. Nuts
5.922	Peanut butter, smooth, USDA Commodity
5.910	Bacon (pork), cured, cooked, pan-fried
5.700	Lima beans, immature, boiled, drained, no salt
5.670	Kellogg's Raisin Bran
5.670	Dark chocolate candies, 60-69% cacao solids (Missing Vitamin Data)
5.650	Cashews, dry roasted, no salt
5.598	McDonald's French Fries
5.502	Potato, Russet, baked, flesh & skin
5.491	Swiss chard, boiled, drained, no salt
5.448	Potato, red, baked, flesh & skin
5.440	Anchovies, European, canned in oil, drained solids
5.360	Banana chips
5.351	Potato, baked, flesh & skin, no salt
5.290	Bay leaf (Missing Data)
5.218	Red snapper, cooked, dry heat
5.151	Soybeans green, boiled, drained, no salt
4.851	Avocado, raw, commercial varieties
4.840	Mushrooms, portabella, raw

4.760	Scallops (bay & sea), steamed
4.750	Sweet potato, baked in skin, no salt
4.661	Spinach, boiled, drained, no salt
4.630	Mace, ground (Missing Data)
4.580	Spearmint, fresh (Missing Data)
4.522	Barley (hulled)
4.410	Walnuts, USDA A259, A257
4.363	Pinto beans, boiled, no salt, mature
4.361	Edamame beans, frozen, prepared
4.340	Whiting, mixed species, cooked in dry heat
4.310	Cinnamon
4.300	Pretzels, hard, whole-wheat (Missing Sugar Data)
4.288	Oats
4.240	Pecans, dry roasted, no salt
4.230	Kraft macaroni & cheese dinner, original, unprepared (Missing Data)
4.210	Pork tenderloin lean, roasted, URMIS 3358
4.070	Chocolate-flavored hazelnut spread (No Trans Fat Data)
4.050	Whole wheat flour
4.028	Kidney beans, red, boiled, no salt, mature seeds
4.007	Garlic, raw
3.951	Avg. Seafood
3.821	Ketchup
3.800	Tilapia, cooked in dry heat
3.779	Salami, dry or hard, pork (No Trans Fat Data)
3.760	Ginger, ground
3.720	Milk chocolate candies (No Trans Fat Data)
3.712	Pak-choi, boiled, drained, no salt
3.692	Lentils, mature seeds, boiled, no salt
3.689	Swordfish, cooked in dry heat
3.640	Puffed Wheat, Quaker
3.629	Macadamia nuts, dry roasted, with salt
3.629	Macadamia nuts, dry roasted, w/out salt
3.581	Banana, raw
3.562	Coconut meat, raw
3.558	Mushrooms, boiled, drained, no salt

3.517	Lobster, northern, cooked in moist heat
3.500	Nutmeg, ground (Missing O3FA Data)
3.441	Flounder (sole), cooked in dry heat
3.415	Avg. Beans & Lentils
3.359	T-bone steak, short loin, beef trimmed to 1/8" fat, all grades, broiled
3.357	Avg. Leafy Green Vegetables
3.350	Velveeta cheese, Kraft, pasteurized spread (Missing Data)
3.310	Tomato sauce, canned
3.300	Bologna, lebanon, beef (No O3FA Data)
3.290	Popcorn, air-popped
3.250	Beets, raw
3.230	Candy bar, Snickers (King Size)
3.203	Carrots, raw, USDA A099
3.140	Whole wheat bread, prepared from recipe
3.130	Bologna, chicken, pork, beef
3.079	Black beans, mature seeds, canned
3.040	Hamburger patty, 80/20 ground chuck beef, broiled
3.040	Sausage, Italian, pork, cooked (No Trans Fat Data)
3.030	Cauliflower, raw
3.019	Avg. Lean Meat
2.950	Basil, fresh
2.929	Broccoli, boiled, drained, no salt
2.920	Turkey, fryer-roaster, breast meat only, roasted
2.909	Chick peas (garbanzo, bengal gram), mature seeds, boiled, no salt
2.900	Rice cakes, brown rice, plain
2.862	Mashed potatoes, home-prepared, whole milk & butter added
2.840	Popcorn, microwave, 94% fat free
2.839	Butternut squash, winter, baked w/out salt, sugar or butter
2.810	Oysters, eastern, wild, cooked, moist heat
2.790	Pepperoni, pork, beef
2.700	Ground turkey, cooked
2.700	Salsa, USDA Commodity (Missing Sugar and Vitamin Data)
2.667	Cantaloupe, raw
2.639	Rye
2.571	Papayas, raw

2.570	Beef sticks, smoked (No Trans Fat Data)
2.560	Blue Cheese (No Trans Fat Data)
2.557	Chicken, broilers or fryers, breast, meat only (no skin), roasted
2.539	Avg. Vegetables
2.528	Zucchini, summer squash, w/ skin, boiled w/out salt, drained
2.480	Whole wheat bread, commecially prepared
2.470	Romaine or cos lettuce
2.460	Horseradish, prepared
2.422	Avg. Cased Meat
2.390	Beef, eye of round, separable lean only, trimmed to 0" fat, all grades, roasted [cube steak]
2.380	Crayfish, mixed species, farmed, cooked in moist heat
2.372	Tuna fish, white, canned in water without salt, drained solids
2.370	Granola bar, soft, uncoated, chocolate chip
2.370	Peanut Butter Cap'n Crunch, Quaker
2.370	Tuna fish, light, canned in water without salt, drained solids
2.369	Tomatoes, raw, red, ripe
2.360	Pomegranate, raw
2.339	Yogurt, regular low-fat, plain, 12 g protein per 8 oz
2.328	Radishes, raw
2.320	FritoLay Sun Chips, Multi-grain snack, original flavor
2.301	Turkey, stuffing, mashed potatoes w/ gravy, assorted vegetables, frozen, microwaved
2.290	Spam, Hormel (Missing Data)
2.277	Kale, boiled, drained, no salt
2.270	Post Honey Bunches of Oats w/ Almonds (Missing Data)
2.250	Teriyaki sauce, ready-to-serve
2.217	Cherries, sweet, raw
2.200	Tortilla chips, plain, yellow corn (Missing Vitamin Data)
2.190	Popcorn, regular butter flavor, microwave, made w/ partially hydrogenated oil (Missing Fats Data)
2.169	Soy sauce (soy & wheat)
2.150	Tortilla chips, plain, white corn
2.122	Corn, sweet, yellow, boiled, drained, no salt
2.107	Peppers, sweet, red, raw
2.100	Pastrami luncheon meat, beef, cured (No Trans Fat Data)
2.040	Syrups, maple

2.022	Asparagus, raw
2.000	Cocoa Puffs, General Mills
1.990	Ice creams, vanilla (No Trans Fat Data)
1.970	Kellogg's Nutri-Grain Cereal Bars, fruit-filled
1.970	McDonald's barbeque sauce
1.970	Cocoa Krispies, Kellogg's (No O3FA Data)
1.960	Cabbage, boiled, drained, no salt
1.907	Grapes, red or green, European type such as Thompson seedless, raw
1.903	Peaches, raw
1.899	Avg. Fruit
1.890	Cheese-flavor puffs or twists, corn-based
1.880	Cap'n Crunch with Crunch Berries, Quaker
1.880	Salami, cooked, beef (No Trans Fat Data)
1.850	Orange, raw, all commercial varieties
1.850	Cap'n Crunch, Quaker
1.820	Lucky Charms, General Mills
1.820	Shrimp, mixed species, cooked in moist heat
1.800	Soy sauce, low sodium (soy & wheat)
1.770	Sesame sticks, wheat-based, salted
1.770	Ice cream, soft-serve, french vanilla (No Trans Fat Data)
1.760	Cake, snack cakes, crème-filled, chocolate with frosting
1.752	Peppers, sweet, green, raw
1.732	Hummus, home prepared
1.730	Ramen noodle soup, chicken flavor, dry
1.721	Chick peas (garbanzo, bengal gram), mature seeds, canned
1.719	Quinoa, cooked
1.700	Whole wheat pita bread
1.660	Milk, nonfat, Ca fortified
1.620	American cheese, pasteurized, w/out disodium phosphate (No Trans Fat Data)
1.600	Chia seeds, dried (Missing Sugar and Vitamin Data)
1.560	Oysters, eastern, wild, raw
1.559	Milk, nonfat, added Vit A
1.558	Mangos, raw
1.544	Slice of pizza, fast food, pizza chain, 14", cheese topping, regular crust (No Trans Fat Data)

1.533	Strawberries, raw
1.520	Cinnamon Toast Crunch cereal, ready-to-eat, General Mills
1.512	Raspberries, raw
1.510	Honey Smacks, Kellogg's
1.500	Milk, lowfat, 1%, added Vit A
1.500	Milk, reduced fat, 2%, added Vit A
1.480	Beets, canned, drained solids
1.468	Cucumber, raw w/ peel
1.464	Snap (green string) beans, boiled, drained, no salt
1.463	Onion, raw
1.460	Acerola (West Indian cherry), raw (Missing Sugar and Vitamin Data)
1.440	Hot Sauce (ready-to-serve, sauce, pepper or hot)
1.430	Milk, whole, 3.25% milkfat
1.410	Iceberg lettuce
1.382	Mustard, prepared, yellow
1.380	Egg, whole, cooked, scrambled
1.379	Cream cheese (No Trans Fat Data)
1.379	Provolone cheese (No Trans Fat Data)
1.360	Pretzels, hard, plain, salted
1.360	Corned beef luncheon meat, beef, cured, canned (No Trans Fat Data)
1.348	Corn chips, extruded, plain
1.332	Brown sugars
1.305	Avg. Cheese
1.300	Hotdog, Oscar Mayer Wiener, beef frank (No Trans Fat Data)
1.288	Mushrooms, canned, drained solids
1.270	Pork-skins, plain
1.250	Golden Crisp, Post, Kraft
1.250	Parmesan cheese, grated (No Trans Fat Data)
1.242	Lemon juice, raw
1.238	Pineapple, canned, juice pack, drained
1.230	Eggplant, boiled, drained, no salt
1.200	White pita bread, enriched
1.200	Honeycomb cereal, Post, Kraft (low data)
1.190	Ritz Crackers, Nabisco (Missing Vitamin Data)
1.172	Mushrooms, shiitake, cooked, no salt

1.168	Spaghetti squash, winter, boiled w/out salt, drained
1.150	Wheat dinner rolls
1.120	Matzo crackers, plain
1.110	Rice Krispies, Kellogg's
1.099	Peas, frozen, boiled, drained, no salt
1.091	Pineapple, raw, all varieties
1.090	Popcorn, caramel-coated without peanuts
1.090	Froot Loops, General Mills
1.080	Roll, hard, kaiser
1.072	White flour, white, all-purpose, enriched, bleached
1.072	Apple, raw, with skin A343
1.070	Apple Jacks, Kellogg's
1.050	Ricotta cheese, whole milk (No Trans Fat Data)
1.040	Grape Juice, canned or bottled, unsweetened
1.012	Wild rice, cooked
1.011	Apple Juice, canned or bottled, unsweetened
1.008	Bagel, plain, unenriched w/ calcium propionate, onion, poppy, sesame (no cream cheese)
1.000	White bread, commercially prepared (inlcudes soft crumbs)
1.000	McDonald's spicy buffalo sauce
0.977	Cheddar cheese (No Trans Fat Data)
0.940	Margarine, industrial, non-dairy, cottonseed, soy oil (partially hydrogenated), for flaky pastries
0.923	Pickles, cucumber, dill or kosher dill
0.881	Pretzels, soft
0.858	Cottage cheese, 1% milkfat (No Trans Fat Data)
0.850	Corn Pops, Kellogg's
0.840	Mozzarella cheese, part skim (No Trans Fat Data)
0.790	Corn Flakes, Kellogg's
0.773	Swiss Cheese (No Trans Fat Data)
0.770	Blueberries, raw
0.770	Apricot jam and preserves
0.760	Mozzarella cheese, whole milk (No Trans Fat Data)
0.732	Instant Oatmeal, Quaker, apples & cinnamon prepared w/ boiling water
0.730	Frosted Flakes, Kellogg's
0.701	Oats, unenriched, boiled, w/out salt

0.621	Millet, cooked
0.560	Parboiled rice, white, long-grain, enriched, cooked
0.519	Honey
0.460	Margarine (vegetable oil spread, 70% fat, soybean & partially hydrogenated soybean, stick)
0.440	Spaghetti, cooked, enriched w/out added salt, no sauce
0.430	Brown rice, long-grain, cooked
0.425	Coffee, brewed from grounds w/ tap water, no sugar or cream (No O3FA Data)
0.420	Olives, pickled, canned or bottled, green
0.400	Light mayo (salad dressing)
0.380	Egg noodles, cooked, enriched
0.370	Black Tea, brewed with tap water
0.350	White rice, long-grain, regular, cooked
0.300	Swanson chicken broth, 99% Fat Free
0.240	Butter, salted (No Trans Fat Data)
0.220	Chicken noodle soup prepared with equal volume water
0.210	Grits, corn, white, regular, quick, enriched, cooked with water, with salt
0.200	Cream of Wheat, instant, prepared with water and salt
0.140	Cranberry juice cocktail, bottled
0.120	Mayonnaise, soybean oil, w/ salt (salad dressing)
0.100	White rice, glutinous, cooked
0.090	Chamomile Tea (No O3FA & O6FA Data)
0.090	White rice, long-grain, pre-cooked or instant, prepared (Missing O3FA Data)
0.080	Salt (table salt)
0.040	Rice noodles, cooked (Missing Sugar & Unsaturated Fat Data)
0.030	Corn starch (Missing O3FA Data)
0.020	Sugars, granulated (sucrose)
0.010	Olive oil (Missing Trans Fat Data)
0.010	Sprite
0.010	Ginger Ale

Sodium

Sodium, mg/SS	Food
387.582	Salt (table salt)
56.369	Soy sauce (soy & wheat)
38.323	Teriyaki sauce, ready-to-serve
36.670	Anchovies, European, canned in oil, drained solids
33.325	Soy sauce, low sodium (soy & wheat)
26.430	Hot Sauce (ready-to-serve, sauce, pepper or hot)
24.280	Bacon (pork), cured, cooked, pan-fried
22.602	Salami, dry or hard, pork (No Trans Fat Data)
21.400	McDonald's spicy buffalo sauce
20.710	Ramen noodle soup, chicken flavor, dry
18.380	Pork-skins, plain
16.530	Pepperoni, pork, beef
15.560	Olives, pickled, canned or bottled, green
15.290	Parmesan cheese, grated (No Trans Fat Data)
14.990	Velveeta cheese, Kraft, pasteurized spread (Missing Data)
14.880	Sesame sticks, wheat-based, salted
14.800	Beef sticks, smoked (No Trans Fat Data)
14.042	Pretzels, soft
13.950	Blue Cheese (No Trans Fat Data)
13.740	Bologna, lebanon, beef (No O3FA Data)
13.690	Spam, Hormel (Missing Data)
13.570	Pretzels, hard, plain, salted
13.510	Carl's Jr. Italian salad dressing, fat free (Missing Data)
12.870	Avg. Cased Meat
12.070	Sausage, Italian, pork, cooked (No Trans Fat Data)
12.000	Mustard, spicy brown, Culver's (Missing Vitamin Data)
11.500	Mustard, Subway, yellow & deli brown (Missing Vitamin Data)
11.400	Salami, cooked, beef (No Trans Fat Data)
11.349	Mustard, prepared, yellow
11.200	Bologna, chicken, pork, beef
11.142	Ketchup
10.250	Hotdog, Oscar Mayer Wiener, beef frank (No Trans Fat Data)
10.170	Cheetos Crunchy cheese-flavored snacks (No O3, 6FA Data)

244

10.100	Chili powder
10.060	Corned beef luncheon meat, beef, cured, canned (No Trans Fat Data)
9.100	Cheese-flavor puffs or twists, corn-based
9.100	McDonald's barbeque sauce
9.070	Rice Krispies, Kellogg's
8.850	Pastrami luncheon meat, beef, cured (No Trans Fat Data)
8.820	Ritz Crackers, Nabisco (Missing Vitamin Data)
8.790	Margarine, industrial, non-dairy, cottonseed, soy oil (partially hydrogenated), for flaky pastries
8.758	Provolone cheese (No Trans Fat Data)
8.748	Pickles, cucumber, dill or kosher dill
8.020	Kraft macaroni & cheese dinner, original, unprepared (Missing Data)
7.710	Popcorn, regular butter flavor, microwave, made w/ partially hydrogenated oil (Missing Fats Data)
7.670	Culver's shrimp cocktail sauce (Missing Vitamin Data)
7.480	Cap'n Crunch, Quaker
7.430	Honeycomb cereal, Post, Kraft (low data)
7.420	Peanut Butter Cap'n Crunch, Quaker
7.320	Bran Flakes, single brand
7.230	Corn Flakes, Kellogg's
7.190	Salsa, Campbell Pace, Thick & Chunky (Missing Vitamin Data)
7.010	Cinnamon Toast Crunch cereal, ready-to-eat, General Mills
7.000	Margarine (vegetable oil spread, 70% fat, soybean & partially hydrogenated soybean, stick)
6.994	Avg. Cheese
6.990	Cap'n Crunch with Crunch Berries, Quaker
6.810	White bread, commercially prepared (inlcudes soft crumbs)
6.790	Lucky Charms, General Mills
6.730	Light mayo (salad dressing)
6.650	Cheerios, General Mills
6.500	American cheese, pasteurized, w/out disodium phosphate (No Trans Fat Data)
6.350	Cocoa Krispies, Kellogg's (No O3FA Data)
6.270	Popcorn, microwave, 94% fat free
6.268	Mozzarella cheese, whole milk (No Trans Fat Data)
6.212	Cheddar cheese (No Trans Fat Data)
6.190	Mozzarella cheese, part skim (No Trans Fat Data)
6.162	Corn chips, extruded, plain

6.071	Monterey Jack cheese (Missing Data)
6.030	Post Honey Bunches of Oats w/ Almonds (Missing Data)
5.800	Kellogg's Raisin Bran
5.758	Butter, salted (No Trans Fat Data)
5.682	Mayonnaise, soybean oil, w/ salt (salad dressing)
5.440	Roll, hard, kaiser
5.360	White pita bread, enriched
5.360	Mayonnaise, Arby's (Missing Vitamin Data)
5.350	Slice of pizza, fast food, pizza chain, 14", cheese topping, regular crust (No Trans Fat Data)
5.344	Bagel, plain, unenriched w/ calcium propionate, onion, poppy, sesame (no cream cheese)
5.330	Cocoa Puffs, General Mills
5.320	Whole wheat pita bread
5.251	Potato chips, plain, salted
5.241	Tomato sauce, canned
5.051	Banquest Hearty Ones Salisbury Steak Dinner w/ Gravy, Mashed Potatoes and Corn in Seasoned Sauce, frozen meal(Missing Data)
4.760	Peanut butter, smooth, USDA Commodity
4.720	Whole wheat bread, commecially prepared
4.710	Froot Loops, General Mills
4.620	Frosted Flakes, Kellogg's
4.520	Parsley, dried (Missing O3FA Data)
4.430	Apple Jacks, Kellogg's
4.300	Salsa, USDA Commodity (Missing Sugar and Vitamin Data)
4.250	Mushrooms, canned, drained solids
4.247	Banquet chicken pot pie, frozen entrée (Missing Data)
4.220	Oysters, eastern, wild, cooked, moist heat
4.210	Tortilla chips, plain, white corn
4.200	Turkey, stuffing, mashed potatoes w/ gravy, assorted vegetables, frozen, microwaved
4.093	Swanson chicken broth, 99% Fat Free
4.062	Cottage cheese, 1% milkfat (No Trans Fat Data)
3.890	Cake, snack cakes, crème-filled, chocolate with frosting
3.860	Corn Pops, Kellogg's
3.842	Black beans, mature seeds, canned
3.736	Avg. Seafood
3.551	New England clam chowder, Campbell's Select (Missing Data)

3.460	Whole wheat bread, prepared from recipe
3.400	Wheat dinner rolls
3.270	FritoLay Sun Chips, Multi-grain snack, original flavor
3.260	Rice cakes, brown rice, plain
3.211	Cream cheese (No Trans Fat Data)
3.171	Mashed potatoes, home-prepared, whole milk & butter added
3.140	Horseradish, prepared
2.992	Chick peas (garbanzo, bengal gram), mature seeds, canned
2.970	Kellogg's Nutri-Grain Cereal Bars, fruit-filled
2.851	Weight Watchers Smart Ones Chicken Enchiladas Suiza, Sour Cream w/ Cheese frozen entrée (Missing Data)
2.810	Tortilla chips, plain, yellow corn (Missing Vitamin Data)
2.800	Egg, whole, cooked, scrambled
2.652	Macadamia nuts, dry roasted, with salt
2.650	Scallops (bay & sea), steamed
2.649	Chicken noodle soup prepared with equal volume water
2.460	Candy bar, Snickers (King Size)
2.430	Cloves, ground
2.419	Hummus, home prepared
2.390	Eggplant, boiled, drained, no salt
2.274	McDonald's French Fries
2.240	Shrimp, mixed species, cooked in moist heat
2.231	Grits, corn, white, regular, quick, enriched, cooked with water, with salt
2.110	Cilantro, dried (No O3FA Data)
2.109	Oysters, eastern, wild, raw
2.080	Dill weed, dried (Missing Data)
2.060	Popcorn, caramel-coated without peanuts
2.030	Pretzels, hard, whole-wheat (Missing Sugar Data)
1.939	Beets, canned, drained solids
1.917	Swiss Cheese (No Trans Fat Data)
1.860	Honey Smacks, Kellogg's
1.790	Granola bar, soft, uncoated, chocolate chip
1.789	Swiss chard, boiled, drained, no salt
1.719	Whey protein powder (Low Data)
1.680	Cumin seed
1.619	Avg. Spice

1.600	Celery seed
1.510	Cream of Wheat, instant, prepared with water and salt
1.500	Golden Crisp, Post, Kraft
1.480	Saffron (Missing Data)
1.320	Whiting, mixed species, cooked in dry heat
1.151	Swordfish, cooked in dry heat
1.120	Clams, mixed species, cooked in moist heat
1.107	Instant Oatmeal, Quaker, apples & cinnamon prepared w/ boiling water
1.070	Ground turkey, cooked
1.047	Flounder (sole), cooked in dry heat
0.970	Crayfish, mixed species, farmed, cooked in moist heat
0.880	Fennel seed (Missing Vitamin & O3FA Data)
0.840	Ricotta cheese, whole milk (No Trans Fat Data)
0.800	Ice creams, vanilla (No Trans Fat Data)
0.800	Mace, ground (Missing Data)
0.792	Milk chocolate candies (No Trans Fat Data)
0.779	Beets, raw
0.770	Marjoram, dried
0.770	Allspice (Missing Data)
0.750	Hamburger patty, 80/20 ground chuck beef, broiled
0.743	Chicken, broilers or fryers, breast, meat only (no skin), roasted
0.720	Avg. Beans & Lentils
0.719	Peas, frozen, boiled, drained, no salt
0.700	Spinach, boiled, drained, no salt
0.698	Yogurt, regular low-fat, plain, 12 g protein per 8 oz
0.690	Carrots, raw, USDA A099
0.670	Fenugreek seed (Missing Vitamin & O3, 6FA Data)
0.659	T-bone steak, short loin, beef trimmed to 1/8" fat, all grades, broiled
0.620	Tarragon, dried (Missing Data)
0.570	Red snapper, cooked, dry heat
0.570	Pork tenderloin lean, roasted, URMIS 3358
0.560	Tilapia, cooked in dry heat
0.560	Salmon, Atlantic, wild, cooked in dry heat
0.553	Avg. Lean Meat
0.550	Potato flour

0.550	Thyme, dried
0.520	Turkey, fryer-roaster, breast meat only, roasted
0.520	Curry powder
0.518	Avg. Leafy Green Vegetables
0.518	Milk, nonfat, Ca fortified
0.500	Tuna fish, light, canned in water without salt, drained solids
0.500	Tuna fish, white, canned in water without salt, drained solids
0.500	Rosemary, dried (Missing Data)
0.440	Black pepper
0.439	Milk, lowfat, 1%, added Vit A
0.420	Milk, nonfat, added Vit A
0.412	Greek yogurt
0.411	Broccoli, boiled, drained, no salt
0.410	Ice cream, soft-serve, french vanilla (No Trans Fat Data)
0.410	Chocolate-flavored hazelnut spread (No Trans Fat Data)
0.410	Milk, reduced fat, 2%, added Vit A
0.400	Apricot jam and preserves
0.400	Milk, whole, 3.25% milkfat
0.390	Radishes, raw
0.384	Avg. Herbs
0.380	Beef, eye of round, separable lean only, trimmed to 0" fat, all grades, roasted [cube steak]
0.380	Turmeric, ground
0.360	Sweet potato, baked in skin, no salt
0.350	Coriander seed (Missing Data)
0.342	Avg. Nuts
0.340	Basil, dried
0.340	Paprika
0.340	Pak-choi, boiled, drained, no salt
0.300	Cauliflower, raw
0.300	Flaxseed
0.300	Spearmint, fresh (Missing Data)
0.280	Brown sugars
0.260	Poppy seed
0.260	Rosemarry, fresh (Missing Data)
0.250	Wheaties, General Mills

0.230	Bay leaf (Missing Data)
0.230	Kale, boiled, drained, no salt
0.211	Avg. Vegetables
0.200	Coconut meat, raw
0.190	Chia seeds, dried (Missing Sugar and Vitamin Data)
0.190	Rice noodles, cooked (Missing Sugar & Unsaturated Fat Data)
0.180	Spaghetti squash, winter, boiled w/out salt, drained
0.180	Cardamom (Missing Data)
0.180	Pumpkin/Squash Seeds, dry roasted, no salt (Missing Vitamin & Se Data)
0.170	Caraway seed
0.170	Lima beans, immature, boiled, drained, no salt
0.170	Garlic, raw
0.160	Anise seed (Missing Sugar, Vitamin, O3FA data)
0.160	Nutmeg, ground (Missing O3FA Data)
0.160	Cashews, dry roasted, no salt
0.160	Cantaloupe, raw
0.150	Oregano, dried
0.140	Potato, Russet, baked, flesh & skin
0.120	Barley (hulled)
0.120	Potato, red, baked, flesh & skin
0.110	Raisins, seedless
0.110	Sage, ground
0.100	Iceberg lettuce
0.100	Pistachio nuts, dry roasted, no salt
0.100	Cinnamon
0.100	Potato, baked, flesh & skin, no salt
0.100	Dark chocolate candies, 60-69% cacao solids (Missing Vitamin Data)
0.099	Pepsi (Missing Data)
0.090	Syrups, maple
0.090	Ginger, ground
0.090	Thyme, fresh (Missing Data)
0.090	Sprite
0.090	Corn starch (Missing O3FA Data)
0.080	Romaine or cos lettuce
0.080	Cabbage, boiled, drained, no salt

0.080	Popcorn, air-popped
0.070	Quinoa, cooked
0.070	Avocado, raw, commercial varieties
0.070	Chick peas (garbanzo, bengal gram), mature seeds, boiled, no salt
0.070	Ginger Ale
0.070	Acerola (West Indian cherry), raw (Missing Sugar and Vitamin Data)
0.060	Peanuts, dry roasted, no salt, all types
0.060	Edamame beans, frozen, prepared
0.060	Mushrooms, portabella, raw
0.060	Banana chips
0.060	Rye
0.050	Tomatoes, raw, red, ripe
0.050	Brown rice, long-grain, cooked
0.050	Grape Juice, canned or bottled, unsweetened
0.050	Whole wheat flour
0.050	Egg noodles, cooked, enriched
0.050	Puffed Wheat, Quaker
0.050	Mustard seed, yellow
0.050	White rice, glutinous, cooked
0.042	Coca Cola Classic
0.040	Peppers, sweet, red, raw
0.040	Oats, unenriched, boiled, w/out salt
0.040	Macadamia nuts, dry roasted, w/out salt
0.040	Honey
0.040	Water, tap, drinking
0.040	Apple Juice, canned or bottled, unsweetened
0.040	Onion, raw
0.040	Mushrooms, shiitake, cooked, no salt
0.040	Basil, fresh
0.040	White rice, long-grain, pre-cooked or instant, prepared (Missing O3FA Data)
0.040	Butternut squash, winter, baked w/out salt, sugar or butter
0.040	Vegetable shortening, household, composite
0.030	Peppers, sweet, green, raw
0.030	Brazil nuts, dried, unblanched
0.030	Papayas, raw

0.030	Zucchini, summer squash, w/ skin, boiled w/out salt, drained
0.030	Pomegranate, raw
0.030	Black Tea, brewed with tap water
0.030	Wild rice, cooked
0.030	Sunflower Seeds, hulled, dry roased, no salt
0.029	Lobster, northern, cooked in moist heat
0.023	Avg. Fruit
0.020	Parboiled rice, white, long-grain, enriched, cooked
0.020	Lentils, mature seeds, boiled, no salt
0.020	Cranberry juice cocktail, bottled
0.020	Asparagus, raw
0.020	Millet, cooked
0.020	Mangos, raw
0.020	White flour, white, all-purpose, enriched, bleached
0.020	Matzo crackers, plain
0.020	High-fructose corn syrup
0.020	Cucumber, raw w/ peel
0.020	Olive oil (Missing Trans Fat Data)
0.020	Mushrooms, boiled, drained, no salt
0.020	Oats
0.020	Grapes, red or green, European type such as Thompson seedless, raw
0.020	Kidney beans, red, boiled, no salt, mature seeds
0.020	Soybeans (aka soy nuts) mature, dry roasted (Missing Sugar and Vitamin Data)
0.020	Walnuts, USDA A259, A257
0.017	Coffee, brewed from grounds w/ tap water, no sugar or cream (No O3FA Data)
0.010	Snap (green string) beans, boiled, drained, no salt
0.010	Pineapple, raw, all varieties
0.010	Banana, raw
0.010	White rice, long-grain, regular, cooked
0.010	Chamomile Tea (No O3FA & O6FA Data)
0.010	Water, bottled, Perrier
0.010	Water, bottled, Poland Spring
0.010	Blueberries, raw
0.010	Pecans, dry roasted, no salt
0.010	Spaghetti, cooked, enriched w/out added salt, no sauce

0.010	Pineapple, canned, juice pack, drained
0.010	Pinto beans, boiled, no salt, mature
0.010	Soybeans green, boiled, drained, no salt
0.010	Strawberries, raw
0.010	Apple, raw, with skin A343
0.010	Lemon juice, raw
0.010	Almonds, USDA A256, A264
0.010	Raspberries, raw

Copper

Copper, mg/SS	Food
0.076	Oysters, eastern, wild, cooked, moist heat
0.044	Oysters, eastern, wild, raw
0.033	Wheaties, General Mills
0.025	Mace, ground (Missing Data)
0.022	Cashews, dry roasted, no salt
0.018	Cilantro, dried (No O3FA Data)
0.018	Sunflower Seeds, hulled, dry roased, no salt
0.017	Brazil nuts, dried, unblanched
0.016	Walnuts, USDA A259, A257
0.016	Poppy seed
0.014	Basil, dried
0.014	Celery seed
0.013	Pistachio nuts, dry roasted, no salt
0.013	Dark chocolate candies, 60-69% cacao solids (Missing Vitamin Data)
0.012	Avg. Nuts
0.012	Pecans, dry roasted, no salt
0.012	Flaxseed
0.011	Soybeans (aka soy nuts) mature, dry roasted (Missing Sugar and Vitamin Data)
0.011	Marjoram, dried
0.011	Black pepper
0.011	Fennel seed (Missing Vitamin & O3FA Data)
0.011	Fenugreek seed (Missing Vitamin & O3, 6FA Data)
0.010	Avg. Herbs
0.010	Coriander seed (Missing Data)
0.010	Nutmeg, ground (Missing O3FA Data)
0.010	Almonds, USDA A256, A264
0.009	Caraway seed
0.009	Cumin seed
0.009	Oregano, dried
0.009	Thyme, dried
0.009	Anise seed (Missing Sugar, Vitamin, O3FA data)
0.009	Mushrooms, shiitake, cooked, no salt
0.008	Curry powder

0.008	Sage, ground
0.007	Avg. Spice
0.007	Clams, mixed species, cooked in moist heat
0.007	Tarragon, dried (Missing Data)
0.007	Pumpkin/Squash Seeds, dry roasted, no salt (Missing Vitamin & Se Data)
0.007	Peanuts, dry roasted, no salt, all types
0.006	Oats
0.006	Macadamia nuts, dry roasted, with salt
0.006	Macadamia nuts, dry roasted, w/out salt
0.006	Bran Flakes, single brand
0.006	Puffed Wheat, Quaker
0.006	Crayfish, mixed species, farmed, cooked in moist heat
0.006	Paprika
0.006	Turmeric, ground
0.006	Thyme, fresh (Missing Data)
0.006	Allspice (Missing Data)
0.006	Parsley, dried (Missing O3FA Data)
0.006	Peanut butter, smooth, USDA Commodity
0.005	Mushrooms, boiled, drained, no salt
0.005	Tortilla chips, plain, white corn
0.005	Chocolate-flavored hazelnut spread (No Trans Fat Data)
0.005	Rosemary, dried (Missing Data)
0.005	Dill weed, dried (Missing Data)
0.005	Barley (hulled)
0.005	Milk chocolate candies (No Trans Fat Data)
0.005	Rye
0.004	Coconut meat, raw
0.004	Whole wheat flour
0.004	Soybeans green, boiled, drained, no salt
0.004	Mushrooms, portabella, raw
0.004	Whole wheat bread, commecially prepared
0.004	Sesame sticks, wheat-based, salted
0.004	Rice cakes, brown rice, plain
0.004	Kellogg's Raisin Bran
0.004	Chili powder

0.004	Mustard seed, yellow
0.004	Basil, fresh
0.004	Bay leaf (Missing Data)
0.004	Cardamom (Missing Data)
0.004	Potato chips, plain, salted
0.004	Chick peas (garbanzo, bengal gram), mature seeds, boiled, no salt
0.003	Salmon, Atlantic, wild, cooked in dry heat
0.003	Edamame beans, frozen, prepared
0.003	Raisins, seedless
0.003	White bread, commercially prepared (inlcudes soft crumbs)
0.003	Whole wheat bread, prepared from recipe
0.003	Whole wheat pita bread
0.003	Cake, snack cakes, crème-filled, chocolate with frosting
0.003	Popcorn, air-popped
0.003	Popcorn, microwave, 94% fat free
0.003	Granola bar, soft, uncoated, chocolate chip
0.003	Scallops (bay & sea), steamed
0.003	Anchovies, European, canned in oil, drained solids
0.003	Cinnamon
0.003	Cloves, ground
0.003	Rosemarry, fresh (Missing Data)
0.003	Saffron (Missing Data)
0.003	Pretzels, hard, whole-wheat (Missing Sugar Data)
0.003	Cocoa Krispies, Kellogg's (No O3FA Data)
0.003	Garlic, raw
0.003	Lima beans, immature, boiled, drained, no salt
0.003	Candy bar, Snickers (King Size)
0.003	Mushrooms, canned, drained solids
0.003	Lentils, mature seeds, boiled, no salt
0.002	Hummus, home prepared
0.002	Avg. Beans & Lentils
0.002	Pinto beans, boiled, no salt, mature
0.002	Avg. Seafood
0.002	Kidney beans, red, boiled, no salt, mature seeds
0.002	Asparagus, raw
0.002	Quinoa, cooked

0.002	Black beans, mature seeds, canned
0.002	Corn chips, extruded, plain
0.002	Pomegranate, raw
0.002	Roll, hard, kaiser
0.002	Wheat dinner rolls
0.002	White pita bread, enriched
0.002	Banana chips
0.002	FritoLay Sun Chips, Multi-grain snack, original flavor
0.002	Pretzels, hard, plain, salted
0.002	Cheerios, General Mills
0.002	Rice Krispies, Kellogg's
0.002	Lucky Charms, General Mills
0.002	Cinnamon Toast Crunch cereal, ready-to-eat, General Mills
0.002	Honey Smacks, Kellogg's
0.002	Golden Crisp, Post, Kraft
0.002	Cap'n Crunch, Quaker
0.002	Peanut Butter Cap'n Crunch, Quaker
0.002	Cap'n Crunch with Crunch Berries, Quaker
0.002	Parmesan cheese, grated (No Trans Fat Data)
0.002	Shrimp, mixed species, cooked in moist heat
0.002	Salami, cooked, beef (No Trans Fat Data)
0.002	Ramen noodle soup, chicken flavor, dry
0.002	Spearmint, fresh (Missing Data)
0.002	Popcorn, regular butter flavor, microwave, made w/ partially hydrogenated oil (Missing Fats Data)
0.002	Post Honey Bunches of Oats w/ Almonds (Missing Data)
0.002	Chia seeds, dried (Missing Sugar and Vitamin Data)
0.002	Avocado, raw, commercial varieties
0.002	Swordfish, cooked in dry heat
0.002	Potato flour
0.002	Salami, dry or hard, pork (No Trans Fat Data)
0.002	Millet, cooked
0.002	Swiss chard, boiled, drained, no salt
0.002	Potato, red, baked, flesh & skin
0.002	Chick peas (garbanzo, bengal gram), mature seeds, canned
0.002	Ketchup

0.002	Spinach, boiled, drained, no salt
0.002	White flour, white, all-purpose, enriched, bleached
0.002	Kale, boiled, drained, no salt
0.002	Bagel, plain, unenriched w/ calcium propionate, onion, poppy, sesame (no cream cheese)
0.002	Sweet potato, baked in skin, no salt
0.001	Mashed potatoes, home-prepared, whole milk & butter added
0.001	Pretzels, soft
0.001	T-bone steak, short loin, beef trimmed to 1/8" fat, all grades, broiled
0.001	Potato, baked, flesh & skin, no salt
0.001	Grapes, red or green, European type such as Thompson seedless, raw
0.001	Egg noodles, cooked, enriched
0.001	Tomato sauce, canned
0.001	Avg. Cased Meat
0.001	Wild rice, cooked
0.001	Mangos, raw
0.001	Pineapple, raw, all varieties
0.001	Peas, frozen, boiled, drained, no salt
0.001	Soy sauce (soy & wheat)
0.001	Soy sauce, low sodium (soy & wheat)
0.001	Zucchini, summer squash, w/ skin, boiled w/out salt, drained
0.001	Pineapple, canned, juice pack, drained
0.001	Teriyaki sauce, ready-to-serve
0.001	Brown rice, long-grain, cooked
0.001	Potato, Russet, baked, flesh & skin
0.001	Blueberries, raw
0.001	Eggplant, boiled, drained, no salt
0.001	Olives, pickled, canned or bottled, green
0.001	Matzo crackers, plain
0.001	Pork-skins, plain
0.001	Ritz Crackers, Nabisco (Missing Vitamin Data)
0.001	Popcorn, caramel-coated without peanuts
0.001	Apricot jam and preserves
0.001	Kellogg's Nutri-Grain Cereal Bars, fruit-filled
0.001	Horseradish, prepared
0.001	Light mayo (salad dressing)

0.001	Corn Flakes, Kellogg's
0.001	Froot Loops, General Mills
0.001	Apple Jacks, Kellogg's
0.001	Cocoa Puffs, General Mills
0.001	Turkey, fryer-roaster, breast meat only, roasted
0.001	Beef, eye of round, separable lean only, trimmed to 0" fat, all grades, roasted [cube steak]
0.001	Pork tenderloin lean, roasted, URMIS 3358
0.001	Hamburger patty, 80/20 ground chuck beef, broiled
0.001	Ground turkey, cooked
0.001	Bacon (pork), cured, cooked, pan-fried
0.001	Tilapia, cooked in dry heat
0.001	Bologna, chicken, pork, beef
0.001	Pepperoni, pork, beef
0.001	Pastrami luncheon meat, beef, cured (No Trans Fat Data)
0.001	Corned beef luncheon meat, beef, cured, canned (No Trans Fat Data)
0.001	Hotdog, Oscar Mayer Wiener, beef frank (No Trans Fat Data)
0.001	Sausage, Italian, pork, cooked (No Trans Fat Data)
0.001	Beef sticks, smoked (No Trans Fat Data)
0.001	Ginger, ground
0.001	Tortilla chips, plain, yellow corn (Missing Vitamin Data)
0.001	Bologna, lebanon, beef (No O3FA Data)
0.001	Spam, Hormel (Missing Data)
0.001	Salsa, USDA Commodity (Missing Sugar and Vitamin Data)
0.001	Acerola (West Indian cherry), raw (Missing Sugar and Vitamin Data)
0.001	Honeycomb cereal, Post, Kraft (low data)
0.001	Slice of pizza, fast food, pizza chain, 14", cheese topping, regular crust (No Trans Fat Data)
0.001	Avg. Lean Meat
0.001	Radishes, raw
0.001	Oats, unenriched, boiled, w/out salt
0.001	McDonald's French Fries
0.001	Raspberries, raw
0.001	Avg. Vegetables
0.001	Chicken noodle soup prepared with equal volume water
0.001	Avg. Leafy Green Vegetables
0.001	Avg. Fruit

0.001	Mustard, prepared, yellow
0.001	Snap (green string) beans, boiled, drained, no salt
0.001	Carrots, raw, USDA A099
0.001	Corn starch (Missing O3FA Data)
0.001	Swiss Cheese (No Trans Fat Data)
0.001	Banana, raw
0.001	Beets, raw
0.001	Cherries, sweet, raw
0.001	Broccoli, boiled, drained, no salt
0.001	Spaghetti, cooked, enriched w/out added salt, no sauce
0.001	Chicken, broilers or fryers, breast, meat only (no skin), roasted
0.001	Lobster, northern, cooked in moist heat
0.001	Beets, canned, drained solids
0.001	Tomatoes, raw, red, ripe
0.001	Peppers, sweet, green, raw
0.001	Instant Oatmeal, Quaker, apples & cinnamon prepared w/ boiling water
0.001	Strawberries, raw
0.001	Spaghetti squash, winter, boiled w/out salt, drained
0.001	Pickles, cucumber, dill or kosher dill
0.001	White rice, long-grain, regular, cooked
0.001	Parboiled rice, white, long-grain, enriched, cooked
0.001	Onion, raw
0.001	Syrups, maple
0.001	Corn, sweet, yellow, boiled, drained, no salt
0.001	Tuna fish, light, canned in water without salt, drained solids
0.001	White rice, long-grain, pre-cooked or instant, prepared (Missing O3FA Data)
0.001	Red snapper, cooked, dry heat
0.001	Tuna fish, white, canned in water without salt, drained solids
0.001	White rice, glutinous, cooked
0.001	Peaches, raw
0.001	Rice noodles, cooked (Missing Sugar & Unsaturated Fat Data)
0.001	Orange, raw, all commercial varieties
0.001	Turkey, stuffing, mashed potatoes w/ gravy, assorted vegetables, frozen, microwaved

Manganese

Manganese, mg/SS	Food
0.300	Cloves, ground
0.284	Saffron (Missing Data)
0.280	Cardamom (Missing Data)
0.175	Cinnamon
0.105	Parsley, dried (Missing O3FA Data)
0.082	Bay leaf (Missing Data)
0.080	Tarragon, dried (Missing Data)
0.079	Thyme, dried
0.078	Turmeric, ground
0.076	Celery seed
0.075	Avg. Spice
0.074	Ginger, ground
0.067	Poppy seed
0.065	Fennel seed (Missing Vitamin & O3FA Data)
0.064	Cilantro, dried (No O3FA Data)
0.056	Black pepper
0.054	Marjoram, dried
0.049	Oats
0.049	Avg. Herbs
0.047	Wheaties, General Mills
0.047	Oregano, dried
0.043	Curry powder
0.039	Pecans, dry roasted, no salt
0.039	Dill weed, dried (Missing Data)
0.038	Whole wheat flour
0.037	Rice cakes, brown rice, plain
0.036	Bran Flakes, single brand
0.034	Walnuts, USDA A259, A257
0.034	Cheerios, General Mills
0.033	Cumin seed
0.033	Syrups, maple
0.032	Basil, dried
0.031	Sage, ground

0.030	Macadamia nuts, dry roasted, with salt
0.030	Macadamia nuts, dry roasted, w/out salt
0.029	Allspice (Missing Data)
0.029	Nutmeg, ground (Missing O3FA Data)
0.028	Kellogg's Raisin Bran
0.027	Pretzels, hard, whole-wheat (Missing Sugar Data)
0.027	Rye
0.025	Flaxseed
0.024	Avg. Nuts
0.023	Almonds, USDA A256, A264
0.023	Anise seed (Missing Sugar, Vitamin, O3FA data)
0.022	Soybeans (aka soy nuts) mature, dry roasted (Missing Sugar and Vitamin Data)
0.022	Chili powder
0.022	Chia seeds, dried (Missing Sugar and Vitamin Data)
0.021	Sunflower Seeds, hulled, dry roased, no salt
0.021	Whole wheat bread, commecially prepared
0.021	Peanuts, dry roasted, no salt, all types
0.020	Puffed Wheat, Quaker
0.020	Barley (hulled)
0.019	Whole wheat bread, prepared from recipe
0.019	Lucky Charms, General Mills
0.019	Rosemary, dried (Missing Data)
0.019	Coriander seed (Missing Data)
0.018	Mustard seed, yellow
0.017	Whole wheat pita bread
0.017	Thyme, fresh (Missing Data)
0.017	Garlic, raw
0.016	Banana chips
0.015	Cinnamon Toast Crunch cereal, ready-to-eat, General Mills
0.015	Mace, ground (Missing Data)
0.014	Rice Krispies, Kellogg's
0.014	Honey Smacks, Kellogg's
0.014	Peanut butter, smooth, USDA Commodity
0.013	Dark chocolate candies, 60-69% cacao solids (Missing Vitamin Data)
0.013	Pistachio nuts, dry roasted, no salt

0.013	FritoLay Sun Chips, Multi-grain snack, original flavor
0.013	Granola bar, soft, uncoated, chocolate chip
0.013	Caraway seed
0.012	Lima beans, immature, boiled, drained, no salt
0.012	Brazil nuts, dried, unblanched
0.012	Fenugreek seed (Missing Vitamin & O3, 6FA Data)
0.012	Brown sugars
0.011	Popcorn, air-popped
0.011	Popcorn, microwave, 94% fat free
0.011	Basil, fresh
0.011	Spearmint, fresh (Missing Data)
0.011	Cocoa Krispies, Kellogg's (No O3FA Data)
0.010	Chick peas (garbanzo, bengal gram), mature seeds, boiled, no salt
0.010	Edamame beans, frozen, prepared
0.010	Wheat dinner rolls
0.010	Clams, mixed species, cooked in moist heat
0.010	Rosemarry, fresh (Missing Data)
0.009	Spinach, boiled, drained, no salt
0.009	Brown rice, long-grain, cooked
0.009	Pineapple, raw, all varieties
0.009	Pretzels, hard, plain, salted
0.009	Sesame sticks, wheat-based, salted
0.009	Chocolate-flavored hazelnut spread (No Trans Fat Data)
0.008	Soybeans green, boiled, drained, no salt
0.008	Cashews, dry roasted, no salt
0.008	Paprika
0.008	Popcorn, regular butter flavor, microwave, made w/ partially hydrogenated oil (Missing Fats Data)
0.007	White flour, white, all-purpose, enriched, bleached
0.007	Matzo crackers, plain
0.007	Cap'n Crunch, Quaker
0.007	Peanut Butter Cap'n Crunch, Quaker
0.007	Oysters, eastern, wild, cooked, moist heat
0.007	Potato chips, plain, salted
0.007	Raspberries, raw
0.006	Quinoa, cooked

0.006	Avg. Beans & Lentils
0.006	Instant Oatmeal, Quaker, apples & cinnamon prepared w/ boiling water
0.006	Froot Loops, General Mills
0.006	Cap'n Crunch with Crunch Berries, Quaker
0.006	Pepperoni, pork, beef
0.006	Oats, unenriched, boiled, w/out salt
0.006	Chick peas (garbanzo, bengal gram), mature seeds, canned
0.006	Hummus, home prepared
0.005	Bagel, plain, unenriched w/ calcium propionate, onion, poppy, sesame (no cream cheese)
0.005	Lentils, mature seeds, boiled, no salt
0.005	Sweet potato, baked in skin, no salt
0.005	White bread, commercially prepared (inlcudes soft crumbs)
0.005	Roll, hard, kaiser
0.005	White pita bread, enriched
0.005	Cake, snack cakes, crème-filled, chocolate with frosting
0.005	Ritz Crackers, Nabisco (Missing Vitamin Data)
0.005	Apple Jacks, Kellogg's
0.005	Cocoa Puffs, General Mills
0.005	Ramen noodle soup, chicken flavor, dry
0.005	Pumpkin/Squash Seeds, dry roasted, no salt (Missing Vitamin & Se Data)
0.005	Milk chocolate candies (No Trans Fat Data)
0.005	Pinto beans, boiled, no salt, mature
0.005	Corn chips, extruded, plain
0.005	Kidney beans, red, boiled, no salt, mature seeds
0.004	White rice, long-grain, regular, cooked
0.004	Soy sauce (soy & wheat)
0.004	Soy sauce, low sodium (soy & wheat)
0.004	Mustard, prepared, yellow
0.004	Tortilla chips, plain, yellow corn (Missing Vitamin Data)
0.004	Strawberries, raw
0.004	Kale, boiled, drained, no salt
0.004	Parboiled rice, white, long-grain, enriched, cooked
0.004	White rice, long-grain, pre-cooked or instant, prepared (Missing O3FA Data)
0.004	Oysters, eastern, wild, raw

0.004	Spaghetti, cooked, enriched w/out added salt, no sauce
0.004	Candy bar, Snickers (King Size)
0.003	Swiss chard, boiled, drained, no salt
0.003	Avg. Leafy Green Vegetables
0.003	Snap (green string) beans, boiled, drained, no salt
0.003	Potato flour
0.003	Egg noodles, cooked, enriched
0.003	Wild rice, cooked
0.003	Raisins, seedless
0.003	Blueberries, raw
0.003	Banana, raw
0.003	Beets, raw
0.003	Slice of pizza, fast food, pizza chain, 14", cheese topping, regular crust (No Trans Fat Data)
0.003	White rice, glutinous, cooked
0.003	Millet, cooked
0.003	Peas, frozen, boiled, drained, no salt
0.003	Beets, canned, drained solids
0.003	McDonald's French Fries
0.003	Black beans, mature seeds, canned
0.002	Grape Juice, canned or bottled, unsweetened
0.002	Potato, baked, flesh & skin, no salt
0.002	Potato, Russet, baked, flesh & skin
0.002	Black Tea, brewed with tap water
0.002	Mushrooms, shiitake, cooked, no salt
0.002	Avg. Fruit
0.002	Cauliflower, raw
0.002	Romaine or cos lettuce
0.002	Cabbage, boiled, drained, no salt
0.002	Popcorn, caramel-coated without peanuts
0.002	Corn Flakes, Kellogg's
0.002	Corn Pops, Kellogg's
0.002	Crayfish, mixed species, farmed, cooked in moist heat
0.002	Butternut squash, winter, baked w/out salt, sugar or butter
0.002	Corn, sweet, yellow, boiled, drained, no salt
0.002	Broccoli, boiled, drained, no salt

0.002	Potato, red, baked, flesh & skin
0.002	Zucchini, summer squash, w/ skin, boiled w/out salt, drained
0.002	Carrots, raw, USDA A099
0.002	Turkey, stuffing, mashed potatoes w/ gravy, assorted vegetables, frozen, microwaved
0.001	Avocado, raw, commercial varieties
0.001	Asparagus, raw
0.001	Avg. Vegetables
0.001	Tomatoes, raw, red, ripe
0.001	Peppers, sweet, green, raw
0.001	Peppers, sweet, red, raw
0.001	Spaghetti squash, winter, boiled w/out salt, drained
0.001	Mushrooms, boiled, drained, no salt
0.001	Onion, raw
0.001	Ketchup
0.001	Tomato sauce, canned
0.001	Pak-choi, boiled, drained, no salt
0.001	Rice noodles, cooked (Missing Sugar & Unsaturated Fat Data)
0.001	Avg. Seafood
0.001	Salt (table salt)
0.001	Pomegranate, raw
0.001	Mushrooms, portabella, raw
0.001	Eggplant, boiled, drained, no salt
0.001	Iceberg lettuce
0.001	Pork-skins, plain
0.001	Cheese-flavor puffs or twists, corn-based
0.001	Horseradish, prepared
0.001	McDonald's barbeque sauce
0.001	Parmesan cheese, grated (No Trans Fat Data)
0.001	Whiting, mixed species, cooked in dry heat
0.001	Anchovies, European, canned in oil, drained solids
0.001	Beef sticks, smoked (No Trans Fat Data)
0.001	High-fructose corn syrup
0.001	Mashed potatoes, home-prepared, whole milk & butter added
0.001	Salami, dry or hard, pork (No Trans Fat Data)
0.001	Honey

0.001	Radishes, raw
0.001	Avg. Cased Meat
0.001	Corn starch (Missing O3FA Data)
0.001	Apple Juice, canned or bottled, unsweetened
0.001	Cherries, sweet, raw
0.001	Lobster, northern, cooked in moist heat
0.001	Cucumber, raw w/ peel
0.001	Grapes, red or green, European type such as Thompson seedless, raw
0.001	Pickles, cucumber, dill or kosher dill
0.001	Mushrooms, canned, drained solids
0.001	Peaches, raw
0.000	Apple, raw, with skin A343
0.000	Chamomile Tea (No O3FA & O6FA Data)
0.000	Chicken noodle soup prepared with equal volume water
0.000	Cranberry juice cocktail, bottled
0.000	Coffee, brewed from grounds w/ tap water, no sugar or cream (No O3FA Data)
0.000	Ginger Ale
0.000	Avg. Cheese
0.000	Orange, raw, all commercial varieties
0.000	Cantaloupe, raw
0.000	Papayas, raw
0.000	Mangos, raw
0.000	Pineapple, canned, juice pack, drained
0.000	Lemon juice, raw
0.000	Coca Cola Classic
0.000	Pepsi (Missing Data)
0.000	Sprite
0.000	Tortilla chips, plain, white corn
0.000	Pretzels, soft
0.000	Apricot jam and preserves
0.000	Kellogg's Nutri-Grain Cereal Bars, fruit-filled
0.000	Hot Sauce (ready-to-serve, sauce, pepper or hot)
0.000	Mayonnaise, soybean oil, w/ salt (salad dressing)
0.000	Light mayo (salad dressing)
0.000	McDonald's spicy buffalo sauce

0.000	Teriyaki sauce, ready-to-serve
0.000	Sugars, granulated (sucrose)
0.000	Golden Crisp, Post, Kraft
0.000	Frosted Flakes, Kellogg's
0.000	Cream of Wheat, instant, prepared with water and salt
0.000	Grits, corn, white, regular, quick, enriched, cooked with water, with salt
0.000	Water, tap, drinking
0.000	Water, bottled, Perrier
0.000	Water, bottled, Poland Spring
0.000	Milk, nonfat, added Vit A
0.000	Milk, nonfat, Ca fortified
0.000	Milk, lowfat, 1%, added Vit A
0.000	Milk, reduced fat, 2%, added Vit A
0.000	Milk, whole, 3.25% milkfat
0.000	Yogurt, regular low-fat, plain, 12 g protein per 8 oz
0.000	Greek style yogurt 150g=2/3 cup (Missing Data)
0.000	Greek yogurt
0.000	Ice creams, vanilla (No Trans Fat Data)
0.000	Ice cream, soft-serve, french vanilla (No Trans Fat Data)
0.000	Margarine (vegetable oil spread, 70% fat, soybean & partially hydrogenated soybean, stick)
0.000	Butter, salted (No Trans Fat Data)
0.000	Cream cheese (No Trans Fat Data)
0.000	Cheddar cheese (No Trans Fat Data)
0.000	Ricotta cheese, whole milk (No Trans Fat Data)
0.000	American cheese, pasteurized, w/out disodium phosphate (No Trans Fat Data)
0.000	Blue Cheese (No Trans Fat Data)
0.000	Swiss Cheese (No Trans Fat Data)
0.000	Provolone cheese (No Trans Fat Data)
0.000	Mozzarella cheese, whole milk (No Trans Fat Data)
0.000	Mozzarella cheese, part skim (No Trans Fat Data)
0.000	Cottage cheese, 1% milkfat (No Trans Fat Data)
0.000	Egg, whole, cooked, scrambled
0.000	Chicken, broilers or fryers, breast, meat only (no skin), roasted
0.000	Turkey, fryer-roaster, breast meat only, roasted

0.000	Beef, eye of round, separable lean only, trimmed to 0" fat, all grades, roasted [cube steak]
0.000	Pork tenderloin lean, roasted, URMIS 3358
0.000	T-bone steak, short loin, beef trimmed to 1/8" fat, all grades, broiled
0.000	Hamburger patty, 80/20 ground chuck beef, broiled
0.000	Ground turkey, cooked
0.000	Bacon (pork), cured, cooked, pan-fried
0.000	Avg. Lean Meat
0.000	Shrimp, mixed species, cooked in moist heat
0.000	Scallops (bay & sea), steamed
0.000	Tuna fish, light, canned in water without salt, drained solids
0.000	Tuna fish, white, canned in water without salt, drained solids
0.000	Salmon, Atlantic, wild, cooked in dry heat
0.000	Tilapia, cooked in dry heat
0.000	Swordfish, cooked in dry heat
0.000	Flounder (sole), cooked in dry heat
0.000	Red snapper, cooked, dry heat
0.000	Salami, cooked, beef (No Trans Fat Data)
0.000	Bologna, chicken, pork, beef
0.000	Pastrami luncheon meat, beef, cured (No Trans Fat Data)
0.000	Corned beef luncheon meat, beef, cured, canned (No Trans Fat Data)
0.000	Hotdog, Oscar Mayer Wiener, beef frank (No Trans Fat Data)
0.000	Sausage, Italian, pork, cooked (No Trans Fat Data)
0.000	Swanson chicken broth, 99% Fat Free
0.000	Olive oil (Missing Trans Fat Data)
0.000	Sesame oil (Missing Trans Fat Data)
0.000	Peanut oil, salad or cooking (No Trans Fat or O3FA Data)
0.000	Palm oil (Missing Trans Fat Data)
0.000	Canola oil (vegetable oil), low erucic acid rapeseed oil
0.000	Grapeseed oil (vegetable oil) (Missing Trans Fat Data)
0.000	Safflower oil (vegetable oil), salad or cooking, linoleic, (over 70%) (No Trans Fat or O3FA Data)
0.000	Sunflower oil (vegetable oil) (Missing Trans Fat & Phytosterol Data)
0.000	Cottonseed (vegetable oil), salad or cooking (Missing Trans Fat Data)
0.000	Corn oil (vegetable oil), industrial and retail, all purpose salad

	or cooking
0.000	Soybean oil, salad or cooking (Missing Phytosterol Data)
0.000	Coconut oil (Missing Trans Fat & O3FA Data)
0.000	Vegetable shortening, household, composite
0.000	Shortening, vegetable, industrial, soy (partially hydrogenated), all purpose
0.000	Margarine, industrial, non-dairy, cottonseed, soy oil (partially hydrogenated), for flaky pastries
0.000	Lard (No Trans Fat Data)
0.000	Mayonnaise, Arby's (Missing Vitamin Data)
0.000	Mustard, spicy brown, Culver's (Missing Vitamin Data)
0.000	Salsa, Campbell Pace, Thick & Chunky (Missing Vitamin Data)
0.000	Culver's shrimp cocktail sauce (Missing Vitamin Data)
0.000	Mustard, Subway, yellow & deli brown (Missing Vitamin Data)
0.000	Carl's Jr. Italian salad dressing, fat free (Missing Data)
0.000	Agave nectar (Missing Data)
0.000	Post Honey Bunches of Oats w/ Almonds (Missing Data)
0.000	Monterey Jack cheese (Missing Data)
0.000	Velveeta cheese, Kraft, pasteurized spread (Missing Data)
0.000	Bologna, lebanon, beef (No O3FA Data)
0.000	Spam, Hormel (Missing Data)
0.000	Kraft macaroni & cheese dinner, original, unprepared (Missing Data)
0.000	Banquet chicken pot pie, frozen entrée (Missing Data)
0.000	New England clam chowder, Campbell's Select (Missing Data)
0.000	Shortening, industrial, soy (partially hydrogenated) for baking & confections (Missing O3FA Data)
0.000	Salsa, USDA Commodity (Missing Sugar and Vitamin Data)
0.000	Acerola (West Indian cherry), raw (Missing Sugar and Vitamin Data)
0.000	Strawberry Jam, Hardee's condiment (Missing Data)
0.000	Cheetos Crunchy cheese-flavored snacks (No O3, 6FA Data)
0.000	Honeycomb cereal, Post, Kraft (low data)
0.000	Whey protein powder (Low Data)
0.000	Weight Watchers Smart Ones Chicken Enchiladas Suiza, Sour Cream w/ Cheese frozen entrée (Missing Data)
0.000	Banquest Hearty Ones Salisbury Steak Dinner w/ Gravy, Mashed Potatoes and Corn in Seasoned Sauce, frozen meal(Missing Data)

Selenium

Selenium, ug/SS	Food
19.173	Brazil nuts, dried, unblanched
1.340	Mustard seed, yellow
1.230	Puffed Wheat, Quaker
0.806	Tuna fish, light, canned in water without salt, drained solids
0.797	Sunflower Seeds, hulled, dry roasted, no salt
0.716	Oysters, eastern, wild, cooked, moist heat
0.707	Whole wheat flour
0.681	Anchovies, European, canned in oil, drained solids
0.657	Tuna fish, white, canned in water without salt, drained solids
0.650	Bacon (pork), cured, cooked, pan-fried
0.640	Clams, mixed species, cooked in moist heat
0.637	Oysters, eastern, wild, raw
0.617	Swordfish, cooked in dry heat
0.582	Flounder (sole), cooked in dry heat
0.544	Tilapia, cooked in dry heat
0.533	Avg. Seafood
0.490	Red snapper, cooked, dry heat
0.486	Honey Smacks, Kellogg's
0.468	Salmon, Atlantic, wild, cooked in dry heat
0.440	Whole wheat pita bread
0.429	Corned beef luncheon meat, beef, cured, canned (No Trans Fat Data)
0.427	Lobster, northern, cooked in moist heat
0.411	Whiting, mixed species, cooked in dry heat
0.410	Pork-skins, plain
0.403	Peanut butter, smooth, USDA Commodity
0.403	Whole wheat bread, commecially prepared
0.396	Shrimp, mixed species, cooked in moist heat
0.391	Roll, hard, kaiser
0.386	Whole wheat bread, prepared from recipe
0.382	Pork tenderloin lean, roasted, URMIS 3358
0.377	Barley (hulled)
0.372	Ground turkey, cooked
0.369	Matzo crackers, plain

0.353	Rye
0.350	Pepperoni, pork, beef
0.342	Crayfish, mixed species, farmed, cooked in moist heat
0.339	White flour, white, all-purpose, enriched, bleached
0.330	Wheat dinner rolls
0.329	Beef, eye of round, separable lean only, trimmed to 0" fat, all grades, roasted [cube steak]
0.329	Mustard, prepared, yellow
0.327	Avg. Lean Meat
0.321	Turkey, fryer-roaster, breast meat only, roasted
0.293	Cilantro, dried (No O3FA Data)
0.293	Parsley, dried (Missing O3FA Data)
0.285	Cheerios, General Mills
0.279	Scallops (bay & sea), steamed
0.276	Chicken, broilers or fryers, breast, meat only (no skin), roasted
0.271	White pita bread, enriched
0.264	Spaghetti, cooked, enriched w/out added salt, no sauce
0.262	Coriander seed (Missing Data)
0.254	Flaxseed
0.254	Salami, dry or hard, pork (No Trans Fat Data)
0.248	Mushrooms, shiitake, cooked, no salt
0.246	Rice cakes, brown rice, plain
0.245	Slice of pizza, fast food, pizza chain, 14", cheese topping, regular crust (No Trans Fat Data)
0.239	Egg noodles, cooked, enriched
0.225	Egg, whole, cooked, scrambled
0.222	T-bone steak, short loin, beef trimmed to 1/8" fat, all grades, broiled
0.220	Sausage, Italian, pork, cooked (No Trans Fat Data)
0.215	Hamburger patty, 80/20 ground chuck beef, broiled
0.211	Avg. Cased Meat
0.193	Soybeans (aka soy nuts) mature, dry roasted (Missing Sugar and Vitamin Data)
0.188	Avg. Spice
0.182	Swiss Cheese (No Trans Fat Data)
0.181	Rice Krispies, Kellogg's
0.177	Parmesan cheese, grated (No Trans Fat Data)
0.177	Pastrami luncheon meat, beef, cured (No Trans Fat Data)

0.173	White bread, commercially prepared (inlcudes soft crumbs)
0.172	Pretzels, soft
0.171	Sesame sticks, wheat-based, salted
0.171	Curry powder
0.170	Mozzarella cheese, whole milk (No Trans Fat Data)
0.164	Lucky Charms, General Mills
0.161	Cocoa Krispies, Kellogg's (No O3FA Data)
0.159	Avg. Nuts
0.157	Bologna, lebanon, beef (No O3FA Data)
0.146	Salami, cooked, beef (No Trans Fat Data)
0.145	Ricotta cheese, whole milk (No Trans Fat Data)
0.145	Blue Cheese (No Trans Fat Data)
0.145	Provolone cheese (No Trans Fat Data)
0.144	American cheese, pasteurized, w/out disodium phosphate (No Trans Fat Data)
0.144	Mozzarella cheese, part skim (No Trans Fat Data)
0.142	Garlic, raw
0.141	Avg. Cheese
0.139	Cheddar cheese (No Trans Fat Data)
0.135	Poppy seed
0.121	Caraway seed
0.121	Celery seed
0.119	Mushrooms, boiled, drained, no salt
0.117	Cashews, dry roasted, no salt
0.117	Macadamia nuts, dry roasted, with salt
0.117	Macadamia nuts, dry roasted, w/out salt
0.115	Hotdog, Oscar Mayer Wiener, beef frank (No Trans Fat Data)
0.111	Granola bar, soft, uncoated, chocolate chip
0.110	Mushrooms, portabella, raw
0.108	Ginger, ground
0.105	Kellogg's Nutri-Grain Cereal Bars, fruit-filled
0.105	Bran Flakes, single brand
0.101	Coconut meat, raw
0.098	Brown rice, long-grain, cooked
0.094	Ramen noodle soup, chicken flavor, dry
0.093	Parboiled rice, white, long-grain, enriched, cooked

0.093	Pistachio nuts, dry roasted, no salt
0.090	Cottage cheese, 1% milkfat (No Trans Fat Data)
0.084	Tortilla chips, plain, yellow corn (Missing Vitamin Data)
0.084	Dark chocolate candies, 60-69% cacao solids (Missing Vitamin Data)
0.083	Corn Flakes, Kellogg's
0.081	Potato chips, plain, salted
0.081	Cheese-flavor puffs or twists, corn-based
0.079	Turkey, stuffing, mashed potatoes w/ gravy, assorted vegetables, frozen, microwaved
0.078	Candy bar, Snickers (King Size)
0.075	Peanuts, dry roasted, no salt, all types
0.075	White rice, long-grain, regular, cooked
0.073	Soybeans green, boiled, drained, no salt
0.069	Popcorn, microwave, 94% fat free
0.069	Cinnamon Toast Crunch cereal, ready-to-eat, General Mills
0.067	Corn chips, extruded, plain
0.067	Tortilla chips, plain, white corn
0.065	Cap'n Crunch, Quaker
0.065	Cocoa Puffs, General Mills
0.065	Corn Pops, Kellogg's
0.063	Fenugreek seed (Missing Vitamin & O3, 6FA Data)
0.062	Pinto beans, boiled, no salt, mature
0.060	Pretzels, hard, plain, salted
0.060	Chili powder
0.059	Froot Loops, General Mills
0.059	Cloves, ground
0.059	Oregano, dried
0.056	Apple Jacks, Kellogg's
0.056	Saffron (Missing Data)
0.056	White rice, glutinous, cooked
0.054	Popcorn, regular butter flavor, microwave, made w/ partially hydrogenated oil (Missing Fats Data)
0.054	Oats, unenriched, boiled, w/out salt
0.052	Cumin seed
0.051	Instant Oatmeal, Quaker, apples & cinnamon prepared w/ boiling water
0.050	Anise seed (Missing Sugar, Vitamin, O3FA data)

0.049	Walnuts, USDA A259, A257
0.048	Chicken noodle soup prepared with equal volume water
0.048	White rice, long-grain, pre-cooked or instant, prepared (Missing O3FA Data)
0.046	Ritz Crackers, Nabisco (Missing Vitamin Data)
0.046	Thyme, dried
0.046	Rosemary, dried (Missing Data)
0.045	Milk chocolate candies (No Trans Fat Data)
0.045	Marjoram, dried
0.045	Turmeric, ground
0.045	Rice noodles, cooked (Missing Sugar & Unsaturated Fat Data)
0.044	Frosted Flakes, Kellogg's
0.044	Tarragon, dried (Missing Data)
0.043	Avg. Herbs
0.041	Mushrooms, canned, drained solids
0.040	Pecans, dry roasted, no salt
0.040	Paprika
0.037	Chick peas (garbanzo, bengal gram), mature seeds, boiled, no salt
0.037	Sage, ground
0.037	Milk, whole, 3.25% milkfat
0.036	Popcorn, caramel-coated without peanuts
0.036	Kellogg's Raisin Bran
0.036	Chocolate-flavored hazelnut spread (No Trans Fat Data)
0.035	Cream of Wheat, instant, prepared with water and salt
0.034	Cake, snack cakes, crème-filled, chocolate with frosting
0.033	Milk, lowfat, 1%, added Vit A
0.033	Yogurt, regular low-fat, plain, 12 g protein per 8 oz
0.031	Milk, nonfat, added Vit A
0.031	Cinnamon
0.031	Black pepper
0.031	Grits, corn, white, regular, quick, enriched, cooked with water, with salt
0.030	Ice cream, soft-serve, french vanilla (No Trans Fat Data)
0.028	Corn starch (Missing O3FA Data)
0.028	Quinoa, cooked
0.028	Horseradish, prepared
0.028	Basil, dried

0.028	Bay leaf (Missing Data)
0.028	Chick peas (garbanzo, bengal gram), mature seeds, canned
0.028	Lentils, mature seeds, boiled, no salt
0.027	Allspice (Missing Data)
0.027	Mace, ground (Missing Data)
0.026	Light mayo (salad dressing)
0.026	Avg. Beans & Lentils
0.025	Almonds, USDA A256, A264
0.025	Milk, reduced fat, 2%, added Vit A
0.024	Cream cheese (No Trans Fat Data)
0.024	Hummus, home prepared
0.023	Asparagus, raw
0.022	Swanson chicken broth, 99% Fat Free
0.021	Milk, nonfat, Ca fortified
0.020	Lima beans, immature, boiled, drained, no salt
0.020	Apricot jam and preserves
0.018	Ice creams, vanilla (No Trans Fat Data)
0.017	Mayonnaise, soybean oil, w/ salt (salad dressing)
0.016	Broccoli, boiled, drained, no salt
0.016	Nutmeg, ground (Missing O3FA Data)
0.015	Spinach, boiled, drained, no salt
0.015	Banana chips
0.013	Black beans, mature seeds, canned
0.012	Kidney beans, red, boiled, no salt, mature seeds
0.011	Potato flour
0.011	Teriyaki sauce, ready-to-serve
0.010	Banana, raw
0.010	Butter, salted (No Trans Fat Data)
0.010	Peas, frozen, boiled, drained, no salt
0.009	Kale, boiled, drained, no salt
0.009	Millet, cooked
0.009	Swiss chard, boiled, drained, no salt
0.009	Avg. Leafy Green Vegetables
0.009	Olives, pickled, canned or bottled, green
0.008	Mashed potatoes, home-prepared, whole milk & butter added
0.008	Potato, red, baked, flesh & skin

0.008	Honey
0.008	Wild rice, cooked
0.008	Soy sauce, low sodium (soy & wheat)
0.007	Beets, raw
0.007	High-fructose corn syrup
0.006	Mangos, raw
0.006	Raisins, seedless
0.006	Radishes, raw
0.006	Cauliflower, raw
0.006	Cabbage, boiled, drained, no salt
0.006	Sugars, granulated (sucrose)
0.006	Acerola (West Indian cherry), raw (Missing Sugar and Vitamin Data)
0.006	Syrups, maple
0.006	Papayas, raw
0.005	Beets, canned, drained solids
0.005	Soy sauce (soy & wheat)
0.005	Potato, Russet, baked, flesh & skin
0.005	Orange, raw, all commercial varieties
0.005	Pomegranate, raw
0.005	Onion, raw
0.005	Butternut squash, winter, baked w/out salt, sugar or butter
0.005	Avg. Vegetables
0.004	Pak-choi, boiled, drained, no salt
0.004	Potato, baked, flesh & skin, no salt
0.004	Romaine or cos lettuce
0.004	Salsa, USDA Commodity (Missing Sugar and Vitamin Data)
0.004	Avocado, raw, commercial varieties
0.004	Strawberries, raw
0.004	Cantaloupe, raw
0.004	Pineapple, canned, juice pack, drained
0.003	Avg. Fruit
0.003	Spaghetti squash, winter, boiled w/out salt, drained
0.003	Basil, fresh
0.003	Cucumber, raw w/ peel
0.003	Ketchup

0.002	Zucchini, summer squash, w/ skin, boiled w/out salt, drained
0.002	Tomato sauce, canned
0.002	Sweet potato, baked in skin, no salt
0.002	Cranberry juice cocktail, bottled
0.002	Lard (No Trans Fat Data)
0.002	Corn, sweet, yellow, boiled, drained, no salt
0.002	Raspberries, raw
0.002	Snap (green string) beans, boiled, drained, no salt
0.001	Grapes, red or green, European type such as Thompson seedless, raw
0.001	Pickles, cucumber, dill or kosher dill
0.001	Pineapple, raw, all varieties
0.001	Apple Juice, canned or bottled, unsweetened
0.001	Peaches, raw
0.001	Salt (table salt)
0.001	Ginger Ale
0.001	Blueberries, raw
0.001	Eggplant, boiled, drained, no salt
0.001	Iceberg lettuce
0.001	Lemon juice, raw
0.001	Carrots, raw, USDA A099
0.001	Peppers, sweet, red, raw

Fluoride

Fluoride, ug/SS	Food
3.730	Black Tea, brewed with tap water
2.339	Raisins, seedless
1.379	Grape Juice, canned or bottled, unsweetened
0.788	Coffee, brewed from grounds w/ tap water, no sugar or cream (No O3FA Data)
0.718	Oats, unenriched, boiled, w/out salt
0.713	Water, tap, drinking
0.689	Ginger Ale
0.672	Cranberry juice cocktail, bottled
0.612	Potato chips, plain, salted
0.562	Grits, corn, white, regular, quick, enriched, cooked with water, with salt
0.559	Sprite
0.520	Corn chips, extruded, plain
0.519	Tortilla chips, plain, white corn
0.489	White bread, commercially prepared (inlcudes soft crumbs)
0.452	Potato, Russet, baked, flesh & skin
0.412	Salami, cooked, beef (No Trans Fat Data)
0.411	White rice, long-grain, regular, cooked
0.378	Spinach, boiled, drained, no salt
0.364	Candy bar, Snickers (King Size)
0.360	Bologna, chicken, pork, beef
0.350	American cheese, pasteurized, w/out disodium phosphate (No Trans Fat Data)
0.349	Cheddar cheese (No Trans Fat Data)
0.349	Tomato sauce, canned
0.342	Black pepper
0.342	Avg. Spice
0.316	Cottage cheese, 1% milkfat (No Trans Fat Data)
0.263	Beets, canned, drained solids
0.233	Avg. Cheese
0.224	Hamburger patty, 80/20 ground chuck beef, broiled
0.203	Pastrami luncheon meat, beef, cured (No Trans Fat Data)
0.195	Avg. Cased Meat
0.186	Tuna fish, light, canned in water without salt, drained solids

0.186	Avg. Seafood
0.186	Rice Krispies, Kellogg's
0.170	Corn Flakes, Kellogg's
0.154	Ice creams, vanilla (No Trans Fat Data)
0.151	Ketchup
0.143	Avg. Leafy Green Vegetables
0.130	Chamomile Tea (No O3FA & O6FA Data)
0.120	Yogurt, regular low-fat, plain, 12 g protein per 8 oz
0.078	Grapes, red or green, European type such as Thompson seedless, raw
0.070	Avocado, raw, commercial varieties
0.070	Spaghetti, cooked, enriched w/out added salt, no sauce
0.070	Honey
0.060	Radishes, raw
0.060	Egg noodles, cooked, enriched
0.050	Milk chocolate candies (No Trans Fat Data)
0.048	Egg, whole, cooked, scrambled
0.044	Strawberries, raw
0.040	Peaches, raw
0.040	Broccoli, boiled, drained, no salt
0.035	Avg. Fruit
0.034	Milk, reduced fat, 2%, added Vit A
0.033	Apple, raw, with skin A343
0.032	Carrots, raw, USDA A099
0.031	Milk, nonfat, added Vit A
0.031	Peanut butter, smooth, USDA Commodity
0.030	Avg. Vegetables
0.028	Butter, salted (No Trans Fat Data)
0.026	Milk, lowfat, 1%, added Vit A
0.023	Cheese-flavor puffs or twists, corn-based
0.023	Tomatoes, raw, red, ripe
0.022	Pinto beans, boiled, no salt, mature
0.022	Banana, raw
0.020	Cherries, sweet, raw
0.020	Peppers, sweet, green, raw
0.020	Salt (table salt)
0.015	Mustard, prepared, yellow

0.013	Cucumber, raw w/ peel
0.011	Onion, raw
0.010	Cauliflower, raw
0.010	Cabbage, boiled, drained, no salt
0.010	Sugars, granulated (sucrose)
0.010	Cantaloupe, raw
0.004	Avg. Beans & Lentils

Zinc

Zinc, mg/SS	Food
1.820	Oysters, eastern, wild, cooked, moist heat
0.907	Oysters, eastern, wild, raw
0.467	Greek style yogurt 150g=2/3 cup (Missing Data)
0.330	Dill weed, dried (Missing Data)
0.170	Cinnamon Toast Crunch cereal, ready-to-eat, General Mills
0.162	Lucky Charms, General Mills
0.161	Cap'n Crunch with Crunch Berries, Quaker
0.160	Cap'n Crunch, Quaker
0.159	Cheerios, General Mills
0.153	Peanut Butter Cap'n Crunch, Quaker
0.125	Cocoa Puffs, General Mills
0.103	Pumpkin/Squash Seeds, dry roasted, no salt (Missing Vitamin & Se Data)
0.079	Poppy seed
0.075	Apple Jacks, Kellogg's
0.075	Cardamom (Missing Data)
0.069	Celery seed
0.062	Hamburger patty, 80/20 ground chuck beef, broiled
0.062	Thyme, dried
0.058	Basil, dried
0.057	Mustard seed, yellow
0.056	Cashews, dry roasted, no salt
0.056	Golden Crisp, Post, Kraft
0.055	Caraway seed
0.053	Sunflower Seeds, hulled, dry roased, no salt
0.053	Anise seed (Missing Sugar, Vitamin, O3FA data)
0.052	Honeycomb cereal, Post, Kraft (low data)
0.051	Pecans, dry roasted, no salt
0.050	Bran Flakes, single brand
0.050	Beef, eye of round, separable lean only, trimmed to 0" fat, all grades, roasted [cube steak]
0.050	Pastrami luncheon meat, beef, cured (No Trans Fat Data)
0.049	Avg. Herbs
0.049	Corn Pops, Kellogg's

0.048	Cumin seed
0.048	Cocoa Krispies, Kellogg's (No O3FA Data)
0.048	Soybeans (aka soy nuts) mature, dry roasted (Missing Sugar and Vitamin Data)
0.047	Froot Loops, General Mills
0.047	Sage, ground
0.047	Cilantro, dried (No O3FA Data)
0.047	Coriander seed (Missing Data)
0.047	Parsley, dried (Missing O3FA Data)
0.047	T-bone steak, short loin, beef trimmed to 1/8" fat, all grades, broiled
0.044	Oregano, dried
0.044	Swiss Cheese (No Trans Fat Data)
0.043	Flaxseed
0.043	Turmeric, ground
0.042	Syrups, maple
0.042	Salami, dry or hard, pork (No Trans Fat Data)
0.041	Kellogg's Nutri-Grain Cereal Bars, fruit-filled
0.041	Curry powder
0.041	Paprika
0.041	Brazil nuts, dried, unblanched
0.040	Oats
0.039	Parmesan cheese, grated (No Trans Fat Data)
0.039	Tarragon, dried (Missing Data)
0.039	Avg. Spice
0.038	Bologna, lebanon, beef (No O3FA Data)
0.037	Rye
0.037	Bay leaf (Missing Data)
0.037	Fennel seed (Missing Vitamin & O3FA Data)
0.036	Bacon (pork), cured, cooked, pan-fried
0.036	Corned beef luncheon meat, beef, cured, canned (No Trans Fat Data)
0.036	Marjoram, dried
0.035	Kellogg's Raisin Bran
0.035	Chia seeds, dried (Missing Sugar and Vitamin Data)
0.034	Avg. Nuts
0.033	Peanuts, dry roasted, no salt, all types
0.033	Provolone cheese (No Trans Fat Data)

0.032	Rosemary, dried (Missing Data)
0.031	Cheddar cheese (No Trans Fat Data)
0.031	Popcorn, air-popped
0.031	Puffed Wheat, Quaker
0.031	Almonds, USDA A256, A264
0.031	Walnuts, USDA A259, A257
0.030	Rice cakes, brown rice, plain
0.030	American cheese, pasteurized, w/out disodium phosphate (No Trans Fat Data)
0.030	Scallops (bay & sea), steamed
0.029	Mozzarella cheese, whole milk (No Trans Fat Data)
0.029	Whole wheat flour
0.029	Ground turkey, cooked
0.029	Avg. Cased Meat
0.028	Popcorn, microwave, 94% fat free
0.028	Mozzarella cheese, part skim (No Trans Fat Data)
0.028	Avg. Cheese
0.028	Barley (hulled)
0.027	Blue Cheese (No Trans Fat Data)
0.027	Clams, mixed species, cooked in moist heat
0.027	Chili powder
0.027	Dark chocolate candies, 60-69% cacao solids (Missing Vitamin Data)
0.027	Peanut butter, smooth, USDA Commodity
0.025	Avg. Lean Meat
0.025	Tortilla chips, plain, white corn
0.025	Pepperoni, pork, beef
0.025	Fenugreek seed (Missing Vitamin & O3, 6FA Data)
0.025	Candy bar, Snickers (King Size)
0.024	Pork tenderloin lean, roasted, URMIS 3358
0.024	Anchovies, European, canned in oil, drained solids
0.024	Sausage, Italian, pork, cooked (No Trans Fat Data)
0.024	Beef sticks, smoked (No Trans Fat Data)
0.024	Potato chips, plain, salted
0.023	Milk chocolate candies (No Trans Fat Data)
0.023	Mace, ground (Missing Data)
0.023	Pistachio nuts, dry roasted, no salt

0.022	Hotdog, Oscar Mayer Wiener, beef frank (No Trans Fat Data)
0.021	Nutmeg, ground (Missing O3FA Data)
0.020	Popcorn, regular butter flavor, microwave, made w/ partially hydrogenated oil (Missing Fats Data)
0.019	Lobster, northern, cooked in moist heat
0.018	Whole wheat bread, commecially prepared
0.018	Salami, cooked, beef (No Trans Fat Data)
0.018	Cinnamon
0.018	Thyme, fresh (Missing Data)
0.018	Velveeta cheese, Kraft, pasteurized spread (Missing Data)
0.018	Spam, Hormel (Missing Data)
0.017	FritoLay Sun Chips, Multi-grain snack, original flavor
0.017	Turkey, fryer-roaster, breast meat only, roasted
0.016	Shrimp, mixed species, cooked in moist heat
0.016	Tortilla chips, plain, yellow corn (Missing Vitamin Data)
0.016	Corn chips, extruded, plain
0.015	Chick peas (garbanzo, bengal gram), mature seeds, boiled, no salt
0.015	Swordfish, cooked in dry heat
0.015	Whole wheat bread, prepared from recipe
0.015	Whole wheat pita bread
0.015	Crayfish, mixed species, farmed, cooked in moist heat
0.014	Pretzels, hard, plain, salted
0.014	Black pepper
0.014	Avg. Seafood
0.014	Slice of pizza, fast food, pizza chain, 14", cheese topping, regular crust (No Trans Fat Data)
0.014	Edamame beans, frozen, prepared
0.013	Wild rice, cooked
0.013	Mushrooms, shiitake, cooked, no salt
0.013	Granola bar, soft, uncoated, chocolate chip
0.013	Rice Krispies, Kellogg's
0.013	Honey Smacks, Kellogg's
0.013	Ginger, ground
0.013	Macadamia nuts, dry roasted, with salt
0.013	Macadamia nuts, dry roasted, w/out salt
0.013	Lentils, mature seeds, boiled, no salt
0.012	Sesame sticks, wheat-based, salted

0.012	Ricotta cheese, whole milk (No Trans Fat Data)
0.012	Bologna, chicken, pork, beef
0.012	Garlic, raw
0.012	Soybeans green, boiled, drained, no salt
0.011	Coconut meat, raw
0.011	Chocolate-flavored hazelnut spread (No Trans Fat Data)
0.011	Cloves, ground
0.011	Spearmint, fresh (Missing Data)
0.011	Saffron (Missing Data)
0.011	Hummus, home prepared
0.011	Quinoa, cooked
0.011	Kidney beans, red, boiled, no salt, mature seeds
0.010	Chick peas (garbanzo, bengal gram), mature seeds, canned
0.010	Cake, snack cakes, crème-filled, chocolate with frosting
0.010	Egg, whole, cooked, scrambled
0.010	Chicken, broilers or fryers, breast, meat only (no skin), roasted
0.010	Post Honey Bunches of Oats w/ Almonds (Missing Data)
0.010	Allspice (Missing Data)
0.010	Pinto beans, boiled, no salt, mature
0.010	Oats, unenriched, boiled, w/out salt
0.010	Avg. Beans & Lentils
0.009	Millet, cooked
0.009	Bagel, plain, unenriched w/ calcium propionate, onion, poppy, sesame (no cream cheese)
0.009	Pretzels, soft
0.009	Roll, hard, kaiser
0.009	Wheat dinner rolls
0.009	Rosemarry, fresh (Missing Data)
0.009	Yogurt, regular low-fat, plain, 12 g protein per 8 oz
0.009	Mushrooms, boiled, drained, no salt
0.008	Salmon, Atlantic, wild, cooked in dry heat
0.008	White pita bread, enriched
0.008	Horseradish, prepared
0.008	Basil, fresh
0.008	Tuna fish, light, canned in water without salt, drained solids
0.008	Spinach, boiled, drained, no salt

0.008	Lima beans, immature, boiled, drained, no salt
0.007	White flour, white, all-purpose, enriched, bleached
0.007	Mushrooms, canned, drained solids
0.007	White bread, commercially prepared (inlcudes soft crumbs)
0.007	Matzo crackers, plain
0.007	Banana chips
0.007	Ice creams, vanilla (No Trans Fat Data)
0.007	Peas, frozen, boiled, drained, no salt
0.006	Avocado, raw, commercial varieties
0.006	Mustard, prepared, yellow
0.006	Flounder (sole), cooked in dry heat
0.006	Egg noodles, cooked, enriched
0.006	Brown rice, long-grain, cooked
0.006	Corn, sweet, yellow, boiled, drained, no salt
0.006	Mushrooms, portabella, raw
0.006	Pork-skins, plain
0.006	Ritz Crackers, Nabisco (Missing Vitamin Data)
0.006	Popcorn, caramel-coated without peanuts
0.006	Ramen noodle soup, chicken flavor, dry
0.006	Pretzels, hard, whole-wheat (Missing Sugar Data)
0.006	Potato flour
0.005	Black beans, mature seeds, canned
0.005	Asparagus, raw
0.005	Cream cheese (No Trans Fat Data)
0.005	Soy sauce (soy & wheat)
0.005	White rice, long-grain, regular, cooked
0.005	Spaghetti, cooked, enriched w/out added salt, no sauce
0.005	Cheese-flavor puffs or twists, corn-based
0.005	Ice cream, soft-serve, french vanilla (No Trans Fat Data)
0.005	Whiting, mixed species, cooked in dry heat
0.005	White rice, long-grain, pre-cooked or instant, prepared (Missing O3FA Data)
0.005	Turkey, stuffing, mashed potatoes w/ gravy, assorted vegetables, frozen, microwaved
0.005	Tuna fish, white, canned in water without salt, drained solids
0.005	Broccoli, boiled, drained, no salt
0.004	McDonald's French Fries

0.004	Red snapper, cooked, dry heat
0.004	Milk, lowfat, 1%, added Vit A
0.004	Milk, reduced fat, 2%, added Vit A
0.004	Milk, whole, 3.25% milkfat
0.004	Milk, nonfat, added Vit A
0.004	Raspberries, raw
0.004	Milk, nonfat, Ca fortified
0.004	Instant Oatmeal, Quaker, apples & cinnamon prepared w/ boiling water
0.004	White rice, glutinous, cooked
0.004	Potato, red, baked, flesh & skin
0.004	Pomegranate, raw
0.004	Tilapia, cooked in dry heat
0.004	Cottage cheese, 1% milkfat (No Trans Fat Data)
0.004	Parboiled rice, white, long-grain, enriched, cooked
0.004	Potato, baked, flesh & skin, no salt
0.004	Beets, raw
0.004	Soy sauce, low sodium (soy & wheat)
0.003	Swiss chard, boiled, drained, no salt
0.003	Avg. Leafy Green Vegetables
0.003	Potato, Russet, baked, flesh & skin
0.003	Avg. Vegetables
0.003	Cauliflower, raw
0.003	Sweet potato, baked in skin, no salt
0.003	Wheaties, General Mills
0.003	Mashed potatoes, home-prepared, whole milk & butter added
0.003	Peppers, sweet, red, raw
0.003	Radishes, raw
0.003	Ketchup
0.002	Raisins, seedless
0.002	Snap (green string) beans, boiled, drained, no salt
0.002	Carrots, raw, USDA A099
0.002	Kale, boiled, drained, no salt
0.002	Rice noodles, cooked (Missing Sugar & Unsaturated Fat Data)
0.002	Honey
0.002	Tomato sauce, canned

0.002	Beets, canned, drained solids
0.002	Tomatoes, raw, red, ripe
0.002	Blueberries, raw
0.002	Iceberg lettuce
0.002	Romaine or cos lettuce
0.002	Cabbage, boiled, drained, no salt
0.002	Light mayo (salad dressing)
0.002	McDonald's barbeque sauce
0.002	Corn Flakes, Kellogg's
0.002	Salsa, USDA Commodity (Missing Sugar and Vitamin Data)
0.002	Cucumber, raw w/ peel
0.002	Cantaloupe, raw
0.002	Spaghetti squash, winter, boiled w/out salt, drained
0.002	Onion, raw
0.002	Mayonnaise, soybean oil, w/ salt (salad dressing)
0.002	Pak-choi, boiled, drained, no salt
0.002	Peaches, raw
0.002	Zucchini, summer squash, w/ skin, boiled w/out salt, drained
0.002	Cream of Wheat, instant, prepared with water and salt
0.002	Chicken noodle soup prepared with equal volume water
0.002	Avg. Fruit
0.001	Banana, raw
0.001	Butternut squash, winter, baked w/out salt, sugar or butter
0.001	Peppers, sweet, green, raw
0.001	Strawberries, raw
0.001	Pickles, cucumber, dill or kosher dill
0.001	Pineapple, raw, all varieties
0.001	Pineapple, canned, juice pack, drained
0.001	Teriyaki sauce, ready-to-serve
0.001	Salt (table salt)
0.001	Eggplant, boiled, drained, no salt
0.001	Apricot jam and preserves
0.001	Hot Sauce (ready-to-serve, sauce, pepper or hot)
0.001	McDonald's spicy buffalo sauce
0.001	Frosted Flakes, Kellogg's
0.001	Margarine (vegetable oil spread, 70% fat, soybean & partially

	hydrogenated soybean, stick)
0.001	Acerola (West Indian cherry), raw (Missing Sugar and Vitamin Data)
0.001	Lard (No Trans Fat Data)
0.001	Butter, salted (No Trans Fat Data)
0.001	Grits, corn, white, regular, quick, enriched, cooked with water, with salt
0.001	Grape Juice, canned or bottled, unsweetened
0.001	Corn starch (Missing O3FA Data)
0.001	Cherries, sweet, raw
0.001	Papayas, raw
0.001	Grapes, red or green, European type such as Thompson seedless, raw
0.001	Mangos, raw
0.001	Orange, raw, all commercial varieties

Phytosterols

Phytosterols, mg/SS	Food
9.679	Corn oil (vegetable oil), industrial and retail, all purpose salad or cooking
8.651	Sesame oil (Missing Trans Fat Data)
4.440	Safflower oil (vegetable oil), salad or cooking, linoleic, (over 70%) (No Trans Fat or O3FA Data)
3.239	Cottonseed (vegetable oil), salad or cooking (Missing Trans Fat Data)
3.130	Cheese-flavor puffs or twists, corn-based
2.560	Cloves, ground
2.440	Sage, ground
2.208	Olive oil (Missing Trans Fat Data)
2.138	Pistachio nuts, dry roasted, no salt
2.050	Peanut oil, salad or cooking (No Trans Fat or O3FA Data)
2.030	Oregano, dried
1.798	Grapeseed oil (vegetable oil) (Missing Trans Fat Data)
1.750	Paprika
1.630	Thyme, dried
1.577	Cashews, dry roasted, no salt
1.552	Avg. Herbs
1.400	Fenugreek seed (Missing Vitamin & O3, 6FA Data)
1.321	Shortening, vegetable, industrial, soy (partially hydrogenated), all purpose
1.260	Avg. Nuts
1.180	Mustard seed, yellow
1.136	Macadamia nuts, dry roasted, with salt
1.136	Macadamia nuts, dry roasted, w/out salt
1.060	Basil, dried
1.007	Avg. Spice
0.920	Black pepper
0.890	Poppy seed
0.858	Coconut oil (Missing Trans Fat & O3FA Data)
0.850	Pecans, dry roasted, no salt
0.830	Chili powder
0.820	Turmeric, ground
0.810	Tarragon, dried (Missing Data)

0.760	Caraway seed
0.730	Mace, ground (Missing Data)
0.720	Curry powder
0.720	Walnuts, USDA A259, A257
0.680	Cumin seed
0.660	Fennel seed (Missing Vitamin & O3FA Data)
0.620	Nutmeg, ground (Missing O3FA Data)
0.600	Celery seed
0.600	Marjoram, dried
0.580	Rosemary, dried (Missing Data)
0.532	Hotdog, Oscar Mayer Wiener, beef frank (No Trans Fat Data)
0.471	Coconut meat, raw
0.471	Sausage, Italian, pork, cooked (No Trans Fat Data)
0.460	Cardamom (Missing Data)
0.460	Coriander seed (Missing Data)
0.440	Rosemarry, fresh (Missing Data)
0.260	Cinnamon
0.250	Beets, raw
0.240	Asparagus, raw
0.232	Ginger, ground
0.180	Cauliflower, raw
0.176	Avg. Cased Meat
0.160	Banana, raw
0.150	Onion, raw
0.149	Avg. Vegetables
0.140	Pickles, cucumber, dill or kosher dill
0.140	Cucumber, raw w/ peel
0.120	Cherries, sweet, raw
0.120	Apple, raw, with skin A343
0.120	Strawberries, raw
0.110	Hummus, home prepared
0.103	Avg. Fruit
0.100	Peaches, raw
0.100	Iceberg lettuce
0.100	Cabbage, boiled, drained, no salt
0.100	Avg. Leafy Green Vegetables

0.100	Spearmint, fresh (Missing Data)
0.100	Cantaloupe, raw
0.090	Horseradish, prepared
0.090	Peppers, sweet, green, raw
0.070	Ketchup
0.070	Radishes, raw
0.070	Tomatoes, raw, red, ripe
0.060	Pineapple, raw, all varieties
0.050	Pepperoni, pork, beef
0.040	Grapes, red or green, European type such as Thompson seedless, raw

Water

Water, g/SS	Food
1.000	Water, tap, drinking
1.000	Water, bottled, Perrier
1.000	Water, bottled, Poland Spring
0.996	Chamomile Tea (No O3FA & O6FA Data)
0.996	Black Tea, brewed with tap water
0.982	Swanson chicken broth, 99% Fat Free
0.957	Radishes, raw
0.956	Iceberg lettuce
0.953	Cucumber, raw w/ peel
0.953	Pak-choi, boiled, drained, no salt
0.950	Zucchini, summer squash, w/ skin, boiled w/out salt, drained
0.946	Tomatoes, raw, red, ripe
0.942	Pickles, cucumber, dill or kosher dill
0.940	Romaine or cos lettuce
0.940	Peppers, sweet, green, raw
0.940	Chicken noodle soup prepared with equal volume water
0.933	Asparagus, raw
0.926	Cabbage, boiled, drained, no salt
0.926	Swiss chard, boiled, drained, no salt
0.923	Avg. Leafy Green Vegetables
0.923	Spaghetti squash, winter, boiled w/out salt, drained
0.921	Basil, fresh
0.919	Peppers, sweet, red, raw
0.919	Cauliflower, raw
0.915	Kale, boiled, drained, no salt
0.914	Acerola (West Indian cherry), raw (Missing Sugar and Vitamin Data)
0.912	Mushrooms, portabella, raw
0.912	Ginger Ale
0.911	Spinach, boiled, drained, no salt
0.910	Mushrooms, boiled, drained, no salt
0.910	Mushrooms, canned, drained solids
0.910	Milk, nonfat, added Vit A
0.910	Tomato sauce, canned

0.908	Beets, canned, drained solids
0.908	Strawberries, raw
0.908	Avg. Vegetables
0.907	Milk, nonfat, Ca fortified
0.906	Lemon juice, raw
0.902	Cantaloupe, raw
0.900	Hot Sauce (ready-to-serve, sauce, pepper or hot)
0.899	Sprite
0.898	Milk, lowfat, 1%, added Vit A
0.897	Eggplant, boiled, drained, no salt
0.897	Salsa, USDA Commodity (Missing Sugar and Vitamin Data)
0.896	Snap (green string) beans, boiled, drained, no salt
0.894	Onion, raw
0.893	Milk, reduced fat, 2%, added Vit A
0.893	Broccoli, boiled, drained, no salt
0.889	Orange, raw, all commercial varieties
0.887	Salsa, Campbell Pace, Thick & Chunky (Missing Vitamin Data)
0.886	Papayas, raw
0.886	Peaches, raw
0.883	Carrots, raw, USDA A099
0.882	Apple Juice, canned or bottled, unsweetened
0.881	Milk, whole, 3.25% milkfat
0.878	Butternut squash, winter, baked w/out salt, sugar or butter
0.875	Beets, raw
0.869	New England clam chowder, Campbell's Select (Missing Data)
0.864	Coffee, brewed from grounds w/ tap water, no sugar or cream (No O3FA Data)
0.862	Cranberry juice cocktail, bottled
0.861	Pineapple, raw, all varieties
0.857	Apple, raw, with skin A343
0.856	Spearmint, fresh (Missing Data)
0.855	Grits, corn, white, regular, quick, enriched, cooked with water, with salt
0.854	Raspberries, raw
0.851	Horseradish, prepared
0.851	Oysters, eastern, wild, raw
0.849	Yogurt, regular low-fat, plain, 12 g protein per 8 oz

0.847	Avg. Fruit
0.846	Grape Juice, canned or bottled, unsweetened
0.842	Cream of Wheat, instant, prepared with water and salt
0.842	Blueberries, raw
0.838	Oats, unenriched, boiled, w/out salt
0.834	Mushrooms, shiitake, cooked, no salt
0.834	Pineapple, canned, juice pack, drained
0.827	Mustard, prepared, yellow
0.823	Cottage cheese, 1% milkfat (No Trans Fat Data)
0.819	Cherries, sweet, raw
0.818	Mangos, raw
0.808	Crayfish, mixed species, farmed, cooked in moist heat
0.808	Grapes, red or green, European type such as Thompson seedless, raw
0.794	Peas, frozen, boiled, drained, no salt
0.785	Instant Oatmeal, Quaker, apples & cinnamon prepared w/ boiling water
0.779	Pomegranate, raw
0.773	Shrimp, mixed species, cooked in moist heat
0.766	Potato, red, baked, flesh & skin
0.764	White rice, glutinous, cooked
0.760	Sweet potato, baked in skin, no salt
0.760	McDonald's spicy buffalo sauce
0.759	Lobster, northern, cooked in moist heat
0.758	Black beans, mature seeds, canned
0.757	Mashed potatoes, home-prepared, whole milk & butter added
0.753	Olives, pickled, canned or bottled, green
0.752	Tuna fish, light, canned in water without salt, drained solids
0.750	Banana, raw
0.749	Potato, baked, flesh & skin, no salt
0.747	Whiting, mixed species, cooked in dry heat
0.746	Potato, Russet, baked, flesh & skin
0.744	Banquest Hearty Ones Salisbury Steak Dinner w/ Gravy, Mashed Potatoes and Corn in Seasoned Sauce, frozen meal(Missing Data)
0.739	Rice noodles, cooked (Missing Sugar & Unsaturated Fat Data)
0.738	Tuna fish, white, canned in water without salt, drained solids
0.738	Wild rice, cooked
0.733	Brown rice, long-grain, cooked

0.731	Flounder (sole), cooked in dry heat
0.731	Avocado, raw, commercial varieties
0.731	Egg, whole, cooked, scrambled
0.729	Edamame beans, frozen, prepared
0.725	Weight Watchers Smart Ones Chicken Enchiladas Suiza, Sour Cream w/ Cheese frozen entrée (Missing Data)
0.721	White rice, long-grain, pre-cooked or instant, prepared (Missing O3FA Data)
0.717	Ricotta cheese, whole milk (No Trans Fat Data)
0.716	Tilapia, cooked in dry heat
0.714	Quinoa, cooked
0.713	Millet, cooked
0.712	Turkey, stuffing, mashed potatoes w/ gravy, assorted vegetables, frozen, microwaved
0.710	Soy sauce, low sodium (soy & wheat)
0.706	Avg. Beans & Lentils
0.706	Soy sauce (soy & wheat)
0.706	Red snapper, cooked, dry heat
0.703	Oysters, eastern, wild, cooked, moist heat
0.703	Parboiled rice, white, long-grain, enriched, cooked
0.697	Lentils, mature seeds, boiled, no salt
0.696	Chick peas (garbanzo, bengal gram), mature seeds, canned
0.695	Corn, sweet, yellow, boiled, drained, no salt
0.695	Pork tenderloin lean, roasted, URMIS 3358
0.695	Pastrami luncheon meat, beef, cured (No Trans Fat Data)
0.692	Ketchup
0.688	Swordfish, cooked in dry heat
0.684	White rice, long-grain, regular, cooked
0.678	Rosemarry, fresh (Missing Data)
0.677	Teriyaki sauce, ready-to-serve
0.675	Egg noodles, cooked, enriched
0.671	Lima beans, immature, boiled, drained, no salt
0.667	Kidney beans, red, boiled, no salt, mature seeds
0.664	Beef, eye of round, separable lean only, trimmed to 0" fat, all grades, roasted [cube steak]
0.664	Avg. Lean Meat
0.658	Bologna, lebanon, beef (No O3FA Data)
0.653	Chicken, broilers or fryers, breast, meat only (no skin), roasted

0.651	Thyme, fresh (Missing Data)
0.650	Hummus, home prepared
0.649	Avg. Seafood
0.644	Turkey, fryer-roaster, breast meat only, roasted
0.641	Banquet chicken pot pie, frozen entrée (Missing Data)
0.636	Clams, mixed species, cooked in moist heat
0.632	Pinto beans, boiled, no salt, mature
0.628	Soybeans green, boiled, drained, no salt
0.621	Spaghetti, cooked, enriched w/out added salt, no sauce
0.610	Ice creams, vanilla (No Trans Fat Data)
0.602	Chick peas (garbanzo, bengal gram), mature seeds, boiled, no salt
0.600	Salami, cooked, beef (No Trans Fat Data)
0.598	Ice cream, soft-serve, french vanilla (No Trans Fat Data)
0.596	Salmon, Atlantic, wild, cooked in dry heat
0.594	Ground turkey, cooked
0.586	Garlic, raw
0.577	McDonald's barbeque sauce
0.577	Corned beef luncheon meat, beef, cured, canned (No Trans Fat Data)
0.564	Bologna, chicken, pork, beef
0.561	Hamburger patty, 80/20 ground chuck beef, broiled
0.559	Light mayo (salad dressing)
0.547	T-bone steak, short loin, beef trimmed to 1/8" fat, all grades, broiled
0.543	Cream cheese (No Trans Fat Data)
0.538	Mozzarella cheese, part skim (No Trans Fat Data)
0.526	Spam, Hormel (Missing Data)
0.517	Avg. Cased Meat
0.503	Anchovies, European, canned in oil, drained solids
0.500	Mozzarella cheese, whole milk (No Trans Fat Data)
0.471	Coconut meat, raw
0.458	Velveeta cheese, Kraft, pasteurized spread (Missing Data)
0.438	Slice of pizza, fast food, pizza chain, 14", cheese topping, regular crust (No Trans Fat Data)
0.437	Avg. Cheese
0.424	Blue Cheese (No Trans Fat Data)
0.409	Provolone cheese (No Trans Fat Data)
0.397	McDonald's French Fries

0.392	American cheese, pasteurized, w/out disodium phosphate (No Trans Fat Data)
0.386	Whole wheat bread, commecially prepared
0.371	Swiss Cheese (No Trans Fat Data)
0.370	Wheat dinner rolls
0.367	Cheddar cheese (No Trans Fat Data)
0.364	White bread, commercially prepared (inlcudes soft crumbs)
0.362	Salami, dry or hard, pork (No Trans Fat Data)
0.345	Apricot jam and preserves
0.327	Whole wheat bread, prepared from recipe
0.326	Bagel, plain, unenriched w/ calcium propionate, onion, poppy, sesame (no cream cheese)
0.321	White pita bread, enriched
0.320	Syrups, maple
0.310	Roll, hard, kaiser
0.307	Pepperoni, pork, beef
0.306	Whole wheat pita bread
0.240	High-fructose corn syrup
0.208	Parmesan cheese, grated (No Trans Fat Data)
0.191	Beef sticks, smoked (No Trans Fat Data)
0.186	Cake, snack cakes, crème-filled, chocolate with frosting
0.171	Honey
0.159	Butter, salted (No Trans Fat Data)
0.158	Margarine, industrial, non-dairy, cottonseed, soy oil (partially hydrogenated), for flaky pastries
0.155	Raisins, seedless
0.150	Pretzels, soft
0.145	Kellogg's Nutri-Grain Cereal Bars, fruit-filled
0.121	Bacon (pork), cured, cooked, pan-fried
0.119	White flour, white, all-purpose, enriched, bleached
0.119	Saffron (Missing Data)
0.114	Turmeric, ground
0.109	Rye
0.106	Cinnamon
0.105	Black pepper
0.103	Whole wheat flour
0.099	Caraway seed

0.096	Barley (hulled)
0.095	Curry powder
0.095	Paprika
0.095	Anise seed (Missing Sugar, Vitamin, O3FA data)
0.093	Rosemary, dried (Missing Data)
0.090	Parsley, dried (Missing O3FA Data)
0.089	Coriander seed (Missing Data)
0.088	Avg. Spice
0.088	Kellogg's Raisin Bran
0.088	Fennel seed (Missing Vitamin & O3FA Data)
0.088	Fenugreek seed (Missing Vitamin & O3, 6FA Data)
0.085	Allspice (Missing Data)
0.084	Corn starch (Missing O3FA Data)
0.083	Cardamom (Missing Data)
0.082	Oats
0.082	Mace, ground (Missing Data)
0.081	Cumin seed
0.080	Sage, ground
0.078	Chili powder
0.078	Thyme, dried
0.077	Kraft macaroni & cheese dinner, original, unprepared (Missing Data)
0.077	Tarragon, dried (Missing Data)
0.076	Marjoram, dried
0.074	Avg. Herbs
0.073	Cilantro, dried (No O3FA Data)
0.073	Dill weed, dried (Missing Data)
0.072	Oregano, dried
0.070	Flaxseed
0.069	Cloves, ground
0.069	Mustard seed, yellow
0.065	Potato flour
0.064	Granola bar, soft, uncoated, chocolate chip
0.064	Basil, dried
0.062	Nutmeg, ground (Missing O3FA Data)
0.060	Celery seed
0.059	Poppy seed

0.058	Rice cakes, brown rice, plain
0.056	Candy bar, Snickers (King Size)
0.054	Bay leaf (Missing Data)
0.049	Chia seeds, dried (Missing Sugar and Vitamin Data)
0.047	Almonds, USDA A256, A264
0.045	Pumpkin/Squash Seeds, dry roasted, no salt (Missing Vitamin & Se Data)
0.043	Matzo crackers, plain
0.043	Banana chips
0.043	Ramen noodle soup, chicken flavor, dry
0.042	Popcorn, microwave, 94% fat free
0.041	Walnuts, USDA A259, A257
0.041	Rice Krispies, Kellogg's
0.039	Pretzels, hard, whole-wheat (Missing Sugar Data)
0.038	Cheerios, General Mills
0.038	Corn Flakes, Kellogg's
0.037	Bran Flakes, single brand
0.037	Puffed Wheat, Quaker
0.035	Brazil nuts, dried, unblanched
0.034	Pretzels, hard, plain, salted
0.033	Popcorn, air-popped
0.033	Frosted Flakes, Kellogg's
0.032	Lucky Charms, General Mills
0.031	Ritz Crackers, Nabisco (Missing Vitamin Data)
0.031	Scallops (bay & sea), steamed
0.030	Froot Loops, General Mills
0.030	Apple Jacks, Kellogg's
0.030	Corn Pops, Kellogg's
0.029	Golden Crisp, Post, Kraft
0.028	Popcorn, caramel-coated without peanuts
0.028	Cocoa Krispies, Kellogg's (No O3FA Data)
0.026	Wheaties, General Mills
0.026	Cinnamon Toast Crunch cereal, ready-to-eat, General Mills
0.026	Ginger, ground
0.026	Popcorn, regular butter flavor, microwave, made w/ partially hydrogenated oil (Missing Fats Data)
0.025	Honey Smacks, Kellogg's

0.025	Cap'n Crunch, Quaker
0.025	Peanut Butter Cap'n Crunch, Quaker
0.025	Cap'n Crunch with Crunch Berries, Quaker
0.023	Tortilla chips, plain, yellow corn (Missing Vitamin Data)
0.023	Potato chips, plain, salted
0.022	Avg. Nuts
0.020	FritoLay Sun Chips, Multi-grain snack, original flavor
0.020	Sesame sticks, wheat-based, salted
0.020	Pistachio nuts, dry roasted, no salt
0.019	Tortilla chips, plain, white corn
0.018	Pork-skins, plain
0.018	Cheese-flavor puffs or twists, corn-based
0.018	Cocoa Puffs, General Mills
0.017	Cashews, dry roasted, no salt
0.016	Macadamia nuts, dry roasted, with salt
0.016	Macadamia nuts, dry roasted, w/out salt
0.016	Peanuts, dry roasted, no salt, all types
0.016	Peanut butter, smooth, USDA Commodity
0.015	Honeycomb cereal, Post, Kraft (low data)
0.015	Milk chocolate candies (No Trans Fat Data)
0.013	Brown sugars
0.013	Dark chocolate candies, 60-69% cacao solids (Missing Vitamin Data)
0.012	Sunflower Seeds, hulled, dry roased, no salt
0.011	Pecans, dry roasted, no salt
0.011	Chocolate-flavored hazelnut spread (No Trans Fat Data)
0.008	Soybeans (aka soy nuts) mature, dry roasted (Missing Sugar and Vitamin Data)
0.004	Corn chips, extruded, plain
0.002	Salt (table salt)

Other Books by the Author

THE GREG DIET: The Busy Person's Answer To Better Health

ALGEBRA IN WORDS – A Guide of Hints, Strategies and Simple Explanations

ALGEBRA IN WORDS 2 – More Hints, Strategies and Simple Explanations

ALGEBRA IN WORDS 3 – Notes for Algebra 2, College Algebra & Pre-Calculus on: Functions, Polynomials, Theorems, Rational Functions & Systems of Equations

Algebra in Words presents: WORD PROBLEMS DECODED

COLLEGE SUCCESS – An Insider's Guide to Higher Grades, More Money, and Better Health

www.ingramcontent.com/pod-product-compliance
Lightning Source LLC
Chambersburg PA
CBHW071149290526
45788CB00001BA/60